January 21st 1974

£3

GUNILLA KNUTSON'S
Book of
Massage

GUNILLA KNUTSON'S
Book of Massage

Illustrations by Rene Moncada

Nelson

Thomas Nelson and Sons Ltd
36 Park Street London W1Y 4DE

PO Box 18123 Nairobi Kenya

Thomas Nelson (Australia) Ltd
597 Little Collins Street Melbourne 3000

Thomas Nelson and Sons (Canada) Ltd
81 Curlew Drive Don Mills Ontario

Thomas Nelson (Nigeria) Ltd

PO Box 336 Apapa Lagos
Thomas Nelson and Sons (South Africa) (Proprietary) Ltd
51 Commissioner Street Johannesburg

First published 1972

0 17 149058 4

Manufactured in the United States of America.

Gunilla Knutson's Book of Massage

A special thanks to George Grenyo for reading my manuscript.

INTRODUCTION

My granduncle arrived in America some fifty years ago. He came from our native Sweden, a country deeply concerned with physical fitness, and he brought with him a special knowledge gained in his youth. He was a masseur.

Today the pace of modern life is frightening. Just trying to live in a natural way makes difficult demands on all of us. To help reduce the strain, any and all means of relaxation are welcome. Sayings such as "You are what you eat," new explorations into vitamins, organic foods, and exercise indicate a feeling for what is going on under the skin.

In one way or another they are all part of the Swedish theory that if you don't feel your best you don't look your best.

That is why I felt the need to write this book. I believe

massage to be an effective method of achieving relaxation through a pleasurable toning and conditioning of the body. In other words, it is a step toward inner peace, an ecology of the spirit. By writing this book I have contributed to the family business in America. But most of all I hope it contributes to your enjoyment of life.

So treat yourself to well-being.

With lots of love, of course.

Gunilla

WHAT IS MASSAGE?

Massage is the manipulation of the tissues and muscles of the body for therapeutic effect. It is a legitimate medical practice, prescribed by doctors for the relief or cure of muscular and organic disorders. Massage can be psychologically as well as physically beneficial. When properly administered it can help relax anyone, no matter how tense or nervous.

Everyone likes to be massaged. Practiced correctly, it has almost an instant soothing effect on aching, overexerted muscles, and it produces a feeling of psychic well-being, which usually continues long after the massage has been completed.

Most people also like to give massages. But there's the rub. There is a great difference between getting a massage and giving one. The receiver of a massage does little but lie still, but the masseur can do real harm if not properly trained. Even a simple "back rub" can cause discomfort or injury if improperly administered.

Massage can become a pleasant addition to the physical life of the healthy individual, relieving minor pains, dispelling fatigue and tension. But first one must have an elementary understanding of the important techniques involved. In this book I will describe the various types and methods of massage, and will offer suggestions on how to use massage for its maximum benefit and enjoyment.

CHAPTER I

A SHORT HISTORY OF MASSAGE

Massage is probably the oldest therapeutic practice known to man. The urge to touch and gently knead or rub a wounded place has always been natural to all human beings. From this instinct a science was gradually developed, and now almost every culture has a traditional style of massage.

Scholars differ on the origin of the word *massage*. Some say it derives from the Greek word *massein* meaning to knead, and was originally applied to the act of washing hair. The Indians used a massage technique known as *tshampua* (shampooing) in their folk medicine, and Alexander the Great enjoyed the services of native masseurs when he stopped in India in 327 B.C. It is thought that members of his army brought the practice back to the Mediterranean, which might explain the

1

similarity in meaning between the Greek and Indian words.

Others trace the word to the Arabic *mass*, which specifically describes the act of massage as "the pressing of the muscular parts of the body in order to give suppleness and stimulate vitality." The precision of this definition proves, these historians claim, that the Arabs invented the practice of massage.

But the ancient Chinese also employed a form of massage so highly developed that it was practiced by a special professional class. When Pehr Henrik Ling developed his system of Swedish gymnastic massage he based it on techniques developed by Kung Foo, a Taoist priest.

No matter who was the first to systematize this animal instinct, the use of massage was highly prevalent in the ancient world. In the *Odyssey,* Homer depicts Greek women rubbing the weary bodies of their returning warriors. Hippocrates, the Greek physician, prescribed massage for treatment of a dislocated shoulder. "Rubbing can bind a joint that is too loose and loosen a joint that is too hard," he wrote. Oriabasus, a Roman physician, described a method of treatment which entailed applying friction to a bruised area, a technique identical to the one used by modern masseurs.

The nontherapeutic benefits of a massage were also known to the ancients. Among the Egyptians, Greeks, Romans and Turks a massage was given after the bath with no other aim but to provide physical pleasure.

The physicians of the Renaissance rediscovered massage in their researches into ancient medical practices. It was used in the sixteenth century to relieve stiffness in joints and muscles. Paracelsus, a Renaissance scholar, further popularized it by describing ancient massage techniques in his book on Egyptian medicine.

The word *massage* first appeared in print in 1818 in a French encyclopedia. Until that time it had been described by its various techniques: rubbing, kneading, palpating, etc. The British referred to it as "medical rubbing" and were the first to use it as a prescribed hospital treatment. In the mid-nineteenth century it became again an accepted medical practice, and its uses were extended to organic and psychic illnesses. Pre-Freudian psychiatrists used massage, in conjunction with hot baths and "rest cures," as therapy for hysteria and severe depression. The extreme asceticism of the Middle Ages did not encourage the physical nature of massage, but some forms of therapeutic massage were probably employed. In the stories of "faith healers" who cured dread diseases and exorcised devils by the "laying on of hands" we can see what might have been a religious justification for the practice of this half-forgotten art. American physicians of the early twentieth century found that massage could relieve the pain and malfunction caused by industrial accidents.

The science of physical therapy was organized around a study of types of massage and their application to a great range of illnesses. Today it is used extensively as a post-operative treatment and is part of the standard regimen prescribed for bed-ridden patients and permanent invalids.

In recent years massage has been discovered to have many nonmedical uses. For those whose psychic tension afflicts their bodies—causing tightness and pain in muscles, head and stomach aches, and inability to function physically—it is the supreme relaxant. Dieters use massage to firm up sagging flesh and maintain muscle tone. Athletes use it after physical exertion to prevent muscle strain and torn and bruised ligaments. Some use it to restore or inspire sexual vigor; others to dispel mental lethargy. In the next chapter I will explain why massage has such a wide range of applications.

CHAPTER II

WHAT MASSAGE DOES

The psychological effects of massage are easy to understand and analyze. Even when a massage is given by a stranger, it is an intimate experience. Massage is usually given in private, and the masseur or masseuse is trained to be gentle, cooperative and amiable. The recipient is made as comfortable as possible, and is aware of the extreme care with which he or she is being treated. No demands are made upon the subject. Nothing is required but total passivity and the acceptance of the masseur's ministrations.

Some professional masseurs have, rightly or wrongly, compared their role to that of a psychologist. They find that after a few sessions many of their clients begin confiding in them, revealing secrets and problems they have kept from their closest friends. Massage loosens inhibitions as well as muscles. The masseur is seen as the most beneficent person in the world, one who brings relief and well-being while making no emotional demands. For those who feel starved of love the masseur is a godsend. Others who just want to be taken care of for a while without the need to reciprocate may occasionally suffer from backaches or headaches, which respond very well to massage.

The physical and psychological benefits of massage are closely linked. Many doctors believe that patients react favorably to massage because of this transmission of "love." For the athlete a brisk massage is a reward for physical exertion as well as a balm for aching muscles. For the dieter a massage often replaces the gratification that was once found in eating. In other words, an effective massage is a combination of physical and psychological factors. It is not just a mechanical process which can be performed by anyone with adequate training. The giver of a massage must be able to communicate concern for the recipient's well-being.

Experiments have shown that massage has a definite physical effect on various parts of the body. The technique of deep kneading, which I will describe later, increases the flow of blood through treated parts and enlarges the small blood vessels (capillaries) to permit greater blood flow through them. This greater circulation can bring relief to an aching limb within a minute or two. It is useless, medically speaking, to continue this type of massage too long, because the blood soon resumes its normal flow. But the psychologically soothing effect of prolonged massage is often a good way to ease tension caused by pain.

The blood itself is affected by massage. The number of red blood cells increases significantly after a period of abdominal stroking, which makes massage helpful in the treatment of some forms of anemia. The blood also develops a greater oxygen capacity, which may be one reason for the increase in physical vigor that some people feel an hour or two after massage.

Lymph glands carry fluid between organs and connective tissues. The rate of flow of this fluid can be accelerated, and made to change direction, by massage. Often when a joint or muscle is inflamed, the lymph glands become obstructed, and fluid does not move freely. Massage can remedy this condition. The squeezing and rolling of the affected muscle is the best way to stimulate lymph flow.

The tranquilizing, soothing action of massage suggests that it does something to the nervous system, although nobody seems to know exactly what. Massage will relieve the pain caused by an inflamed or severed nerve, but the nature of its interaction with nerve impulses remains a mystery.

Massage is the most effective means of restoring an aching or weary muscle to normal performance. Muscle cramps or spasms respond immediately to forceful kneading. Muscular vigor is revived even after an exhausting day of hard physical work. You can perform a muscle massage on yourself and feel its results in minutes. Do a series of arm exercises—pushups. Massage the muscles you have used and rest for a while. Then do those same exercises again. You will find that the fatigue caused by the original exertion has been almost totally removed by the massage. But if you had merely rested between exercise bouts, you would be stiff and unable to perform. Massage must be used in conjunction with exercise to restore tone and strength to muscles. What it does is enable the muscle to strengthen itself by providing greater mobility and stamina for exercise.

Skin tone and texture are improved by the technique of stroking. Blood circulation through the blood vessels under the skin is increased, and sweat glands are opened, permitting greater secretion of waste and old tissue.

These are some of the things massage can do. It is thought that certain techniques may also have a beneficial effect on bone structures, metabolism, and kidneys, gall bladder and other visceral organs. Physical therapists massage the abdominal area to relieve constipation. Forceful kneading of the lower back while the patient is in a prone position may lessen severe gastric pains in some instances. But massage is not generally recommended as a cure for discomfort or illness in visceral regions. It is used in the treatment of bone fractures because physicians believe that increased blood circulation speeds healing. But this is a highly therapeutic type of massage and should not be attempted by amateurs.

Here are some of the things massage definitely *cannot* do:

It cannot stimulate hair growth. There are many variations of scalp massage, many miracle treatments that promise to produce a luxuriant growth on a bald pate within weeks. Sad to say, none of them has proven successful. Baldness is transmitted genetically. It can be avoided only by synthetic means, a wig or transplants.

Massage cannot restore sexual potency. Male impotence and female frigidity are psychological conditions, which might be relieved by the soothing, anxiety-dispelling action of a massage, but not by any physical effect. A person with serious sexual inhibitions will not be helped by massage.

Massage is not a wonder cure to be taken in isolation without the necessity for any other activity. It is most effective when combined with exercise, good diet and a receptive mental attitude.

CHAPTER III

THE TIME AND THE PLACE

I spent a large portion of my early years as a model "on the road." During one particular promotion tour I ended up in Chicago after several very tiring days of television appearances and modeling assignments. When I arrived at the hotel I was tense and tired from the traveling, and I wanted to unwind. So I called down and made an appointment with the house masseur. I thought that a massage would put me in a relaxed frame of mind for the TV show I had to appear on in less than two hours.

Very wrong!

There is a time and a place for everything, and massage is no exception. As I remember it, "The Chicago Massage" relaxed me so thoroughly that I could hardly stay awake, much less be charming and eloquent on the show!

So you see, both body and mind are more receptive to

the benefits of massage at certain times of the day, and before or after certain activities. There are certain times when a massage is not only useless, but even irritating or counterproductive. There are certain environments in which massage should not be performed. Where massage is concerned, knowing where and when is just as important as knowing how.

The recipient must be able to focus mental and physical attention on the massage in order for it to be a pleasurable and effective experience. The actual hour of the day is not the deciding factor, but rather what mental and physical activities have preceded and will follow the massage.

Never sandwich a massage in between appointments. If the recipient knows there is a limited amount of time available, complete relaxation will be impossible. Impatience and anxiety about being on time will override everything. A person on a tight schedule should make massage the last order of business for the day. Businessmen who go for a workout and massage in the middle of the day, and then jump right back into the rat race, deprive themselves of the full benefits of the experience. The worst place to be a clock watcher is on the massage table, so leave yourself plenty of time to relax. The same holds true for the giver of a massage. Patience and concentration are the key attributes of a good masseur; impatience and distraction make the experience practically useless.

A massage after a meal will confuse the system, interfering with digestion and producing more discomfort than anything else. Why is the system confused? Directly after a meal large quantities of blood circulate around the stomach to help begin the digestive process. If, at the same time, a counterprocess is begun which seeks to detour the blood away from its destination and circulate it faster around inactive parts, discomfort results.

Massage directly before a meal is also not advisable. A body in need or anticipation of nourishment can never be fully relaxed, and several minutes of strenuous activity on both the giver's and receiver's parts will be wasted. Often the hunger-weakened subject will be reduced to exhaustion by this further claim on his body.

Massage is invigorating, but not to a person who wants nothing more than a few hours' sleep. Fatigue is best cured by rest. In its weakened state the fatigued body may be harmed by a vigorous massage.

Similarly, the body that has just performed strenuous physical exercise should not be immediately massaged. Athletes do not run to the training table right after a game. They shower and rest for a while before a massage to give their muscles a chance to dissipate some of the mental and physical tension that exercise builds up.

Never try to cure a serious injury with massage. Only a cramp or spasm will respond well to kneading without risk of aggravation. Sprains, torn ligaments, broken or fractured bones and dislocations should be treated by a physician.

Now, when are the best times to massage? First, when the need and desire are consciously felt. When the recipient has nothing else to think about and wants nothing more than a massage, that is certainly the best time to give it. This might occur after a relaxing, sedentary day at the beach, or maybe on a Sunday afternoon when the most strenuous activity of the day has been lifting the Sunday paper. After a bath or shower, both body and mind are receptive to a vigorous working-over. And, of course, a massage is the perfect end to a few hours in a health club. If taken in combination with a steam bath and a cold shower, it will make the body sing with health and vigor.

Psychologically, massage is emotional compensation and reinforcement. It is the perfect tonic for frustration or anxiety. It can act as an emotional reward for strenuous mental work that perhaps has not yet borne fruit. The famous "hard day at the office," which so often produces fatigue and depression, can be forgotten after a few minutes of massage. Suddenly decisions don't seem so crucial; fears and antagonisms are put in perspective; inhibitions are released. But do not overestimate the psychological benefits of massage. They provide temporary relief at best. The recipient must be mentally conditioned to massage. He or she must have had it under non-stress circumstances, must know what to expect from it and how to react.

The environment in which a massage is given is another crucial factor. Our responses to the same experience will vary with the setting and atmosphere. Most people get the maximum benefits from massages that are given in private, quiet surroundings. The experience is an extremely personal one, involving an intimate physical relationship between two people. The rapport that is established can be shattered easily by an interruption from the outside world.

It is for this reason that massage is enjoyed best in the privacy of the home. I have seen people being massaged on public beaches, in full view of hundreds of people. But I think they are more concerned with telling the world something about themselves—that they are free spirits or are very much in love, or whatever message they think a massage communicates to an onlooker—than with actually enjoying the experience.

A serious massage should be given in a quiet room without any distractions (soft music, perhaps, if it helps the recipient to relax, but that is all). The room should be comfortably warm; if the body is cold, the muscles will contract and will not respond readily. Odors, intrusive sounds and sights should be eliminated. Don't go to extremes and seal off a room for massage, but be aware that little distractions can diminish the effect. Exceptions can be made. If the recipient likes to watch television or is relaxed by loud, blaring music, and the masseur can stand it also, then by all means let it blare. But the object is to create a perfect setting, and this depends on the people involved.

A premium massage table is the best place to get and give a massage, but most homes are not equipped with one. The next best thing is a good bed with a firm mattress and a backboard. A floor covered with a fairly thick carpet is also a good place. (A bare wooden floor might be too cold and uncomfortable.) The object is to find a surface that will provide maximum support and comfort while keeping the body horizontal. During the warm seasons a secluded spot in the outdoors can make a pleasant setting. If your surface is grass, be sure the ground is level. If the body is placed in an unnatural position—on a slight incline or a bumpy surface—the massage will be uncomfortable and possibly harmful. Massages given on the beach, even over a thick blanket, are never too successful because of the uneven surface of the sand. This is not to say that they cannot be pleasant, but that there are better places and circumstances.

As you will see, massage techniques vary in effect and difficulty of execution. Some are very demanding on giver and recipient. Others are casual, providing a moment's transitory comfort, and not meant to have lasting effect. You can lie in a smoke-filled room with the television on and get a good deal of gratification from having your back scratched. This, however, is not a massage. Those who make massage a part of their regular routines quickly learn how crucial a little care in the selection of time, place and circumstance can be.

CHAPTER IV

THE COMPLEAT MASSEUR

Basically, the good masseur has four attributes:

1. Physical strength, especially in hands, fingers and shoulders
2. Physical cleanliness
3. Solid knowledge of the human anatomy
4. A healthy mental attitude

Three of these four can be easily developed with a little study and care. The fourth, mental attitude, is dependent upon the masseur's attitude toward the recipient. Professionals, of course, are motivated mainly by a pride in their craft, a desire to please the recipient to insure further patronage.

Now, how strong do you have to be? The brute force of a weightlifter isn't necessary. But a masseur has to be able to perform such actions as pushing, kneading, deep stroking and hammering over a fairly long period of time. Five to ten minutes may not seem that long, but when you are doing constant physical labor it is not inconsiderable. Women (and men too!) may find it congenial to strengthen the fingers and wrists by kneading dough. This exercise, performed ten to fifteen minutes at a time, is surprisingly demanding to untrained hands, but it can be very effective in developing massaging muscles. Piano playing helps too.

Getting your arms and shoulders in shape is a simple matter. A few minutes of pushups and/or chins should suffice. If you can do ten pushups or five chins, then you have the necessary endurance for giving a massage.

Your hands and fingers must be strong but sensitive, a very difficult combination to achieve. A masseur's fingers probe the body for sensitive areas, feeling out weaknesses and treating them. There are several ways to strengthen the fingers. If you're really ambitious, try fingertip pushups. Get in the standard pushup position, but instead of placing your palms on the floor, balance yourself on your fingers and do the exercise. This is extremely difficult for people of normal strength. Consider yourself more than adequate if you can do five of these.

Another way to strengthen the fingers is to lift various objects with them. Make pincers out of your fingers, close them over the object and lift. You won't find this too easy either. One hand is stronger than the other in most people; this inequality in strength extends to the fingers also. The ring finger and pinky are usually weaker than the other three. The inequality should be eliminated as much as possible, or an unequal intensity of massage pressure will result. Remember, the massage recipient should be completely unaware of the presence of hands after the massage has begun. This state is difficult to achieve if pressure and force are not evenly distributed.

In the hands, the grip must be strengthened. The best way to do this is to buy a pair of nutcracker grips in an athletic supply store, and to begin by seeing how many times in a row you can squeeze them shut. Some of these devices demand more arduous labor than others, but anywhere from fifteen to twenty-five squeezes in succession will be more than enough. You can perform the same exercise with a hard rubber ball, only the number of squeezes should be multiplied at least ten times.

Your fingers will become sensitive with experience. Just like the baker who can tell if bread is done by touching it, or an experienced shopper who can distinguish ripe from rotten fruit with a few squeezes, you will also learn to think with your fingers. You can prepare yourself a little by becoming familiar with the touch of your own body. Run your fingers up and down your arms, chest and legs. Get the feel of the hillocks of muscle, the hard expanses of bone. See if you can locate the beginning and end of your ribcage.

Try to visualize what the various anatomical structures look like in the body, and how they respond to manipulation. The action of massage has been compared to squeezing a tube until it's empty. You've seen this done, you've done it yourself. Now close your eyes and try to visualize this process of extrusion being repeated in the blood and lymph vessels of the body. Kneading muscles has been compared to molding hard clay. While kneading your own arm or leg muscles, try to visualize what this does to the body. Constant practice with the fingers will soon establish a rapport between brain and fingertips.

Soon you will be unconsciously, almost instinctively, thinking with your fingers.

The hands of a masseur must be totally relaxed; the slightest bit of tension will be immediately communicated to the recipient. The relaxation must be mental and physical. The mental I will discuss later.

There are two very simple exercises to prepare the hands physically. Ball your hands into fists and hold them clenched tightly for as long as you can. Then unclench and straighten your fingers, stretching them. After you've done this several times, let your hands drop limply from your wrists and shake them vigorously. When you stop you'll feel a slight vibration in your palms from the quickened flow of your blood. Your hands and fingers should be relaxed and limber; you are physically ready to give a massage.

In such an intimate experience as massage, personal cleanliness on the part of the giver and the recipient is a must. The masseur's hands must be especially cared for. They should be smooth, soft and free of calluses. If you have naturally dry skin, apply a light coating of skin cream after you wash your hands. Keep your nails short and smooth. Rings, bracelets, watches, and other objects likely to get in your way should be removed.

Study the diagrams on the following pages. It isn't necessary to memorize every muscle and nerve in the body. You should only be concerned with getting a general idea of what the anatomical structures are and how they link up with one another. Many of us have the feeling that our bodies are made of isolated islands of muscle and organ. Massage would not be half so effective if that were the case. Our physical components act together and depend on each other. This helps explain why headaches are sometimes caused by back trouble and can be cured by spinal massage. Many other conditions and sensations originate in one part of the body and are felt in another. Learning something about the structure and texture of the parts of the body affected by massage will help you understand why the various massage techniques are effective in their different ways.

And now for the mental attitude. In the process of massage the giver and the recipient must have complementary expectations. The recipient expects some form of gratification, in the form of relief or pleasure. The giver should actively want to supply this gratification. Otherwise, the massage will not be successful and shouldn't be given.

If you, as the masseur, don't look forward to your task, then don't perform it. Never give a massage mechanically, without enthusiasm, just because you've been asked to do so. Never give one when you're angry with the recipient, or if you're just indifferent. You must want the recipient to feel pleasure as much as he or she wants to. Otherwise your indifference or hostility will be communicated, your casual attitude will be interpreted as hostility, and the whole experience will become very unpleasant.

You have to enjoy being a masseur, enjoy the physical contact involved. If you're an amateur, you must have enough feeling for the recipient to enjoy giving pleasure. People who give massages only in the hopes of getting massaged in return almost never do a very good job.

CHAPTER V

MASSAGE TECHNIQUES

Although there are as many different types of massage as there are different cultures, they all make use of the same basic techniques. Each stroke or technique has its own effect and has to be performed at a certain rate of speed for a given length of time. These basic techniques are *petrissage, kneading, friction, effleurage* and *tapotement.*

PETRISSAGE

This technique, used primarily in Swedish massage, combines the motions of kneading and rolling. It is used as a muscle relaxer and conditioner. It is executed by lifting a piece of muscle away from the bone, holding it between the fingers and thumbs of both hands, and rolling it between the fingers, allowing small portions of the muscle to slip through the fingers back to the bone. This maneuver should be repeated on an area of the muscle adjacent to the one which has just been treated. The whole muscle is massaged in this manner. If the flesh is plentiful, the muscle can be held between the palms of the hands and kneaded slowly. Pressure should be firm, but not enough to cause discomfort.

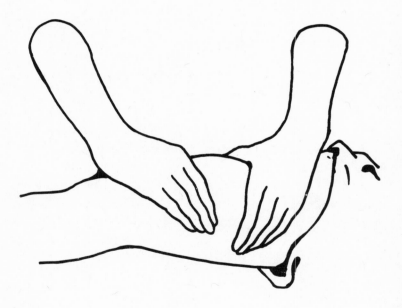

Petrissage is best performed on the larger muscle groups of the back, arms and legs. It causes a sudden infusion of blood into the massaged tissue, which in turn speeds healing or cell nourishment, as well as providing a relaxing effect. Petrissage is an excellent tension remover, especially for people whose anxiety expresses itself in stiff and aching muscles.

KNEADING

The technique of kneading is based on the same principle as petrissage, but the application is slightly different. The palms of the hands are placed on either side of the area to be massaged. With very gentle pressure, the flesh is kneaded in slow, circular movements, with the palms working in opposite directions. The pressure exerted varies with the part being massaged. "Superficial" or light kneading is used on tissue just below the skin. "Deep" or heavy kneading is used when a specific muscle is the object.

Kneading can also be performed on smaller areas by grasping the flesh with the palms and kneading with the thumbs. Aside from its relaxing effect, it also helps to cure sudden muscle spasms in the legs, arms or shoulders.

FRICTION

This movement involves deep rubbing with the palms over large anatomical areas. Most masseurs agree that the pressure applied should be heavy. Some like to begin

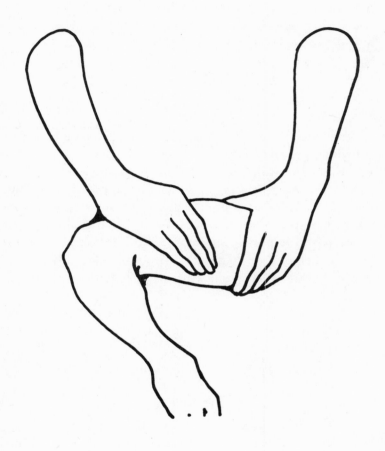

lightly, gently stroking the skin and then pressing more deeply. Others believe that the slight shock engendered by an immediately heavy touch is beneficial. Friction is performed by placing the palms flat on the skin and making circular motions which increase in radius as the massage progresses. Some masseurs apply friction with the fingertips alone, but the pressure is never as uniform as when done with the whole palm.

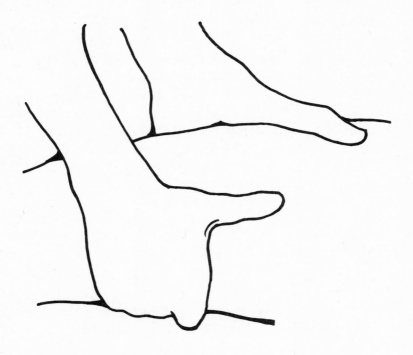

Deep friction moves the subcutaneous (under the skin) tissues over the larger ones directly below them. It stimulates the flow of blood through the subcutaneous capillaries, producing a tingling effect and soothing minor pains on nerves and muscles.

EFFLEURAGE

This movement is performed by stroking the body in the direction of the blood currents in the veins, in other words, toward the heart. The stroking can be done with any part of the hand, depending upon the desired effect. When done with the heel or palm, the effect of friction is simulated; when done with the fingers, the balls of the thumbs or the knuckles, the action is somewhat similar to kneading. The pressure exerted in this movement varies also with the purpose of the massage. For therapeutic purposes the pressure can be as heavy as possible.

TAPOTEMENT
(Judo Chop)

The vision most uninformed people have of a massage is of a burly masseur grinning sadistically and pounding some poor person senseless with a series of judo chops. Needless to say, this is a bit exaggerated. When properly performed, the tapotement technique is one of the most relaxing of all the massage movements. The shock that is experienced upon receiving tapotement does not lead to pain or discomfort, but to greater conditioning of the treated

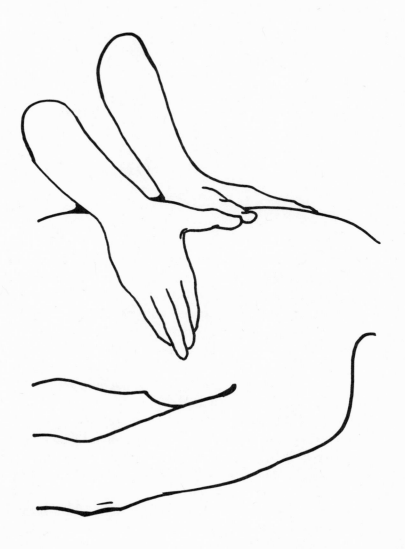

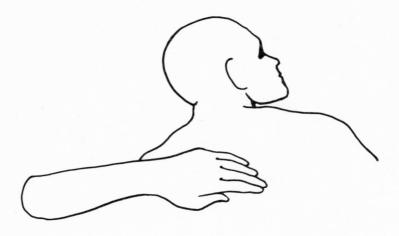

parts. Tapotement is an integral part of Swedish and Japanese massage and is used as the *coup de grace* or culmination of the treatment.

To execute this movement, hold your fingers together and extend them as far as they will go. This is the judo chop position. Bring your palms together and begin striking the area that is being massaged with each hand. Alternating your hands, strike rapidly, keeping your blows close together so that the entire area is covered. If your palms rub against each other as you strike, you will know that no fragment of skin is being left untouched. Move from one end of the area to the other. When you have reached the end, return to where you started and begin again.

The blows should bounce off the skin in a staccato pattern. They should be firm but not excessively so. A good way to gauge firmness is by the reaction of the recipient's body. If it involuntarily recoils under the blows, then you are striking too hard. The recipient may moan and groan, but if the body remains motionless under this rain of blows, you will know that they are not causing real pain or damage.

Swedish masseurs sometimes cup the hands slightly and strike with the palms. This softens the impact of the blow considerably, and may be used on especially sensitive areas of the body around the neck and spine. Chiropractors use variations of the chop to shock the patient into relaxation and to realign the spinal column. Without warning they deliver a sharp blow to the neck right at the top of the spine. This causes momentary mental confusion; most patients also break into a cold sweat. The maneuver is repeated sporadically whenever the spine has fallen out of alignment.

Athletes often use tapotement to condition the muscles of the abdomen. They lie on their backs with their feet lifted just enough to tense the stomach muscles. A masseur then delivers a barrage of judo chops on the abdominal muscles, striking with as much force as the recipient can bear. This maneuver is repeated on a daily basis until the recipient can tolerate blows of considerable force without recoiling.

Tapotement should not be administered at the beginning of a massage. The muscles have not been adequately prepared for its shock effect and will not respond. Common sense should tell you those places where it should never be used. The face, head, Adam's apple, collar bone, breasts and genitals are definitely off-limits for this technique.

There are many variations of these basic massage

movements. Stroking, especially, has been broken down into sensual techniques. Among them are the *consecutive fingertip maneuver,* in which the fingers play lightly along the flesh, as if performing a glissando on the keys of a piano; the *circular vibrating technique* involving gentle circular stroking with the fingertips; and the *fingernail technique,* movement using light stroking pressure from the fingernails along the body's erogenous zones. These are nontherapeutic techniques and can be used only for superficial relaxation or as components of sexual play.

Massage movements cannot be performed properly without careful attention to the pressure exerted, the rhythm of the strokes or movements, the direction of the movements, condition of the skin and the frequency of massage.

Masseurs should follow Hippocrates' dictum in regard to pressure: "Hard rubbing binds; soft rubbing loosens; much rubbing causes parts to waste; moderate rubbing makes them grow." The pressure exerted should relate to the aim of the massage. In most cases you will want to relax the recipient and to condition normal muscles. Thus, most amateurs should use soft to moderate pressure, never succumbing to the temptation to knead too firmly or strike too vigorously.

There should be a consistent rhythmic pattern to a massage. The number of movements per minute should be uniform, and the body should be handled as if in time with a piece of music. The speed of treatment varies with the movement. Tapotement should be administered as quickly as possible without losing control over the amount of force. Effleurage or stroking is done slowly for maximum effect, and petrissage should be given at a consistent, moderate pace. Do not vary the speed of a movement once you have begun it. Consistency is the best way to stimulate relaxation and conditioning.

The direction of the movement should be centripetal or toward the center. This means that when you're kneading or stroking in a circular pattern, do it toward the center of that circle. Always move toward the center of the body and the heart, except when performing light effleurage, in which case you can stroke away from the heart at the beginning, but change direction as you increase pressure.

Do not abuse the skin to amuse the muscles. Naturally dry skin can become severely irritated as the result of a vigorous massage. Remember, the earliest writers on the subject included the process of "anointing" as one of the chief components of massage. Olive oil was a favorite balm of the ancients and for a while was thought to have curative properties of its own. Some kind of liquid or cream is needed for any sustained massage. The choice is a matter of mutual taste. Baby oil, cold cream, petroleum jelly, lanolin, cocoa butter and alcohol are among the many possibilities. An alcohol rub is very effective for reconditioning exerted muscles. When worked into the skin it creates a feeling of spreading warmth. Other creams and oils help keep the massage surface lubricated. They should be applied sparingly, just enough to cover the area. You want your hand to slide, not slip over the skin.

You can give or get massages as often as you wish. The frequency of massage is only regulated in therapeutic instances. Some variations of Swedish and Japanese massage are very demanding, and they can begin having a detrimental effect if given too often. But this is entirely a matter of individual taste. You should be the best authority on the condition of your own body. If you are sore after a massage, feel more tense and stiff than when you began, you are obviously indulging too much. Unlike exercise, massage is not supposed to leave the muscles sore and weary; it is supposed to banish such conditions. Unlike medication, massage is not something one must have daily to restore health. Don't get the idea that a daily massage is obligatory. It will be effective only if you are looking forward to it.

CHAPTER VI

WAYS OF MASSAGING DIFFERENT BODY PARTS

Not every part of the body can be massaged in the same manner. It wouldn't be productive to deliver a series of judo chops to the head; nor is it necessary to be particularly gentle when stroking the upper back. Some muscles respond to pressure, others don't. Each part of the body has different sensitivities and needs different treatment.

HEAD

Let's start at the top. Most people don't think of the head as being a fit subject for massage. But for those whose tension manifests itself in headaches and stiffness of the neck, massage is the only nonchemical answer.

The recipient lies prone (face downward) and the

masseur takes a position directly over the head. The fingers are placed gently at the base of the neck just above the spinal column, and a circular vibrating movement is begun toward the top of the skull. The hands move upward, but the pressure exerted is downward toward the neck and spine. As you move farther up the head, reduce the pressure slightly until it is at its lightest in the area around the temples. When the top of the skull is reached, the movement can be repeated from its starting point.

A particularly effective variation is to place the index and middle fingers of one hand together at the point where the neck joins the skull. Vibrate your arm as if you were shivering, while maintaining a steady, light pressure.

Such movements are effective in relieving tension headaches, and this is a good way to begin a whole body massage. In many people the upper regions of the body, the head and neck, are repositories of the tension which is felt lower down in the back and limbs. Massaging the head in the manner described above often helps relax these lower areas.

A scalp massage can be quite restful, although it will not stimulate hair growth. Again, begin at the base of the neck, this time a little lower down on the back. Use the circular vibrating technique, but this time keep the touch lighter, the movements faster, and direct the pressure up toward the scalp. When the top of the skull is reached, reverse direction, heading down to the neck, but keeping the pressure moving up toward the skull. Vigorous rubbing or friction of the scalp produces pleasurable sensations for some people, but it does not stimulate the flow of blood to that region, nor does it relax the head muscles.

In other variations of head massage the recipient lies

supine (face upward), and the masseur stands directly over the head so that his hands can reach the massaged area without reaching or straining.

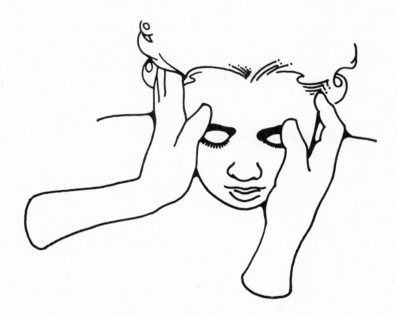

Slow, gentle digital (finger) kneading along the front part of the head sometimes relieves aches in the temples and forehead region. Place your thumbs on the temples and spread your fingers wide enough to cover the area from the top of the ears to just below the scalp. Knead the head with the fingers, using slow circular movements until the entire head has been covered. Do not lift your fingers to change position, but slide them slightly along. Release pressure before changing your position or you will pull the hair along with you. When the entire head has been covered, the movement can be repeated from the starting point. Pressure should be as heavy as possible without causing discomfort. This is one massage you can perform effectively on yourself.

FACE

Facial massage is both therapeutic and cosmetic. It is used with great success in the treatment of insomnia and headaches. In conditioning the facial muscles, it prevents the formation of wrinkles, improves muscle tone and keeps facial skin looking fresh and youthful.

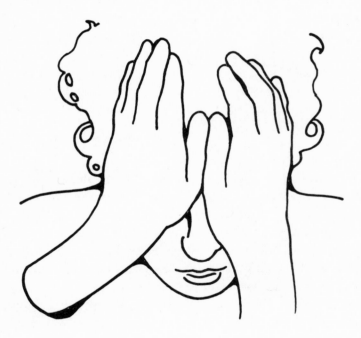

In facial massage the recipient lies supine, with the masseur standing directly over the face. One technique that relieves tension headaches in the temples and forehead is gentle or "superficial" stroking of that region with the palms. Place the palms next to one another on the forehead, the fingers bent slightly to grasp the head. With a very light touch, stroke out toward the edges of the forehead, keeping the fingers on the head, the palms sliding up and down the massaged area. When the outer borders of the forehead have been reached, assume the original position and begin again.

This same movement can be performed over the cheeks by lowering the position of the palms to the cheekbones and keeping the fingers lightly anchored to the forehead. Also stroke slowly and gently to the outer edge of the cheeks and perform the movement again from the original position.

Although small in total area, the face has many places which can be massaged. Each of the features responds to concentrated treatment, and the larger areas like the forehead, cheeks and chin can also be separately massaged. But before treating the separate parts it is good practice to perform a total facial massage. This is best done with light circular stroking. Place the index and middle fingers of each hand on the recipient's temples. Stroking slowly and in a circular pattern, move horizontally across the forehead. Then change direction, moving vertically up from the bridge of the nose. Cover the entire forehead with tiny, gentle, circular strokes. Then move down to the eyes, the nose, the ears and, finally, place your fingers at each end of the jawbone below each ear and work your way down to the chin, where your fingers will meet.

Throughout this movement the pressure should be exerted downward in the direction of the throat and neck. The strokes should be leisurely and light, and the entire treatment should take a minimum of five minutes. This is another type of massage you can perform on yourself. It can be done lying in bed, in a bath, or sitting at the breakfast table. It is a quick, superficial relaxer, so don't

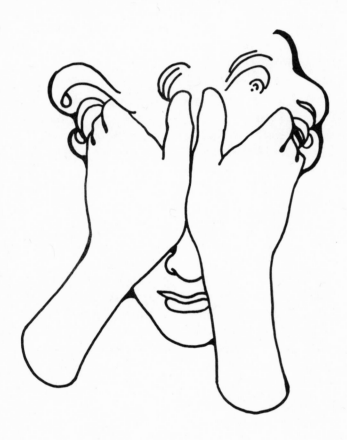

count on it to relieve headaches or sinus troubles. There are other movements for that.

Deep stroking of the forehead and temples can simply melt away certain types of head pain if properly done. Grasp your subject's forehead with the palms, the way you would a basketball, with the thumbs coming together at the hairline. Now stroke laterally toward the edge of the forehead. Be firm but not excessive. Try to stretch the skin so that the recipient's eyes must close. Don't rub. Stroke in one direction. If you feel great resistance from the skin,

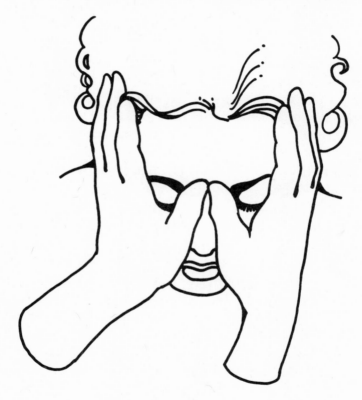

you'll know you're pressing too hard. When you reach the edge of the forehead, return to the original position and repeat this movement twice.

Sinus headaches, eyestrain and general tension in the area around the eyes and nose can also be relieved by deep stroking. Place the thumbs together at the tip of the nose with the fingers at the temples and begin kneading up toward the bridge of the nose. When your thumbs reach the valleys between the eyes and the nose, stop kneading and make deep strokes with the thumbs heading upward over the eyebrows and out toward the temples. Return your thumbs to their original positions and repeat this movement four or five times.

Now place the fingers on the temples and the thumbs in the hollows under the eyes. You will feel a bone structure under your thumbs. This is the infra-orbital ridge. Stroke over that ridge to the tips of the eyebrows. Then return to the original position and repeat the movement three or four times.

Stroking seems to wipe or melt tension away. Kneading gives the illusion of seeking it out from between the crevices in bone and muscle, patiently working it away until not a trace remains. Place the fingertips at the temples and the thumbs over the bridge of the nose. Knead upward in small circles to the hairline. Then return to a slightly different position at the lower border of the forehead and repeat the movement, going upward and returning to a different spot until the entire forehead has been covered.

Kneading downward from temples to neck or shoulders is another effective movement. Bunch your fingers at the temples and knead in small circles back over the hairline and along the backs of the ears until the fingers meet at the cervical vertebra, which is located just above the neck. Resume the original position and repeat this movement once. Then place the fingers at the temples again, but this time knead over the fronts of the ears, down the neck to the tips of the shoulders, repeating this movement once. Do not perform the same movement over and over again because the recipient says it feels good. The law of diminishing returns will begin to apply, and soon the movement will lose its effectiveness, and, if continued after that, it could cause discomfort.

Gentle kneading with the palms can be applied to various areas of the face. Cup your palms over the cheeks, letting your fingers rest lightly on the forehead. Knead in large circles, three times in a forward direction, three times in a backward direction. Keep the palms from moving over the skin. Only the skin over the cheekbone should be in motion. Do this movement twice.

NECK

I've always held that if lack of time prevents you from getting a complete massage and that only one part of the body can be massaged that part should be the neck.

Famous jazz harpist Corky Hale agrees with me and feels that after hours of practicing nothing relaxes her more than a neck rub. She says that her husband, songwriter Mike Stoller ("Is That All There Is," "Kansas City" and a flock of Elvis Presley tunes) is a super neck manipulator. The collarbone has not produced a hit tune yet but it has provided many lyrical moments!

The neck is very sensitive in its front part and capable

of absorbing vigorous manipulation in its back. You must use different movements and pressure in massaging it.

Gentle manipulation of the front part of the neck should begin the massage. The recipient is supine, and the masseur stands directly over the neck, usually to the right. The index and middle fingers are placed behind the earlobes and with light circular stroking are worked down the sternocleidomastoid muscles to the collarbone. Then the fingers are positioned in front of the ear lobes and worked down between the sternocleidomastoids and the Adam's apple. Repeat this movement, this time gently stroking the area around the windpipe. This technique, in combination with certain facial movements, is used in the treatment of insomnia.

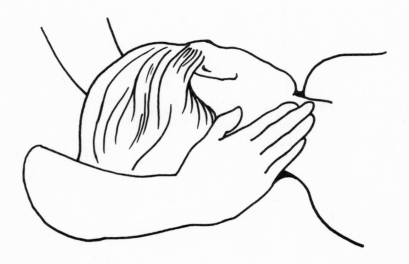

To continue the neck massage, petrissage is done on the sternocleidomastoid muscles, beginning at the collarbone and continuing up to the skull. Keep the manipulation gentle and stop as soon as the recipient feels the slightest discomfort. You may have to ask if any pain is being felt, because some people think that pain is an inevitable companion of massage and shouldn't even be mentioned. Now repeat the stroking maneuvers, only in reverse—beginning with the windpipe, then the area between the Adam's apple and the sternocleidomastoids and then those muscles themselves. Be aware that you are dealing with the recipient's breathing apparatus and keep your pressure suitably light.

When these movements have been completed, have the recipient roll into a prone position, face downward, arms at sides. Lightly stroke the back of the neck, using the circular vibrating technique. Now, beginning at the base of the skull, move down to the top of the spine with heavier stroking movements, exerting pressure down toward the spine. Do this until the entire neck has been covered. When the recipient is tense, the trapezius muscles at the base of the neck are hard and unyielding to the touch. Continue this stroking, intensifying the pressure slightly, until these muscles soften and become more pliable. Then repeat the entire movement from the beginning, expanding the circular strokes and lightening the pressure. If the stroking technique has relaxed the trapezius muscles, you can then perform vigorous petrissage on them, following the course of the muscles from the base of the skull to the upper back. Tapotement can also be applied to the trapezius muscles, but only if much of the tension has been demonstrably relieved by the other movements. Do not attempt to relax a rigid, tense muscle with the judo chop technique.

You can gauge the amount of suitable pressure from the physical condition of the recipient. Active, athletic people have well-developed back and neck muscles. The trapezius muscles are among the strongest in the body and can absorb a good deal of pressure. An athletic man, for example, could take almost the full force of your strength in the stroking movement and in petrissage too. But do not hasten the application of heavy pressure. The recipient's muscles must show some reaction to light stroking before the more vigorous movement begins. When repeating the movement, keep the pressure light, even if the recipient has not complained of pain. This repetition is a reinforcement of the benefits of the original movement, not an exact duplicate of it.

The trapezius muscles are the key to the relaxation of the head, neck and shoulders. There are three special techniques for the massage of these muscles alone.

1. The thumbs touch the bottom borders of the trapezium, with the palms meeting on the tops of the shoulders. The hands move upward, but stroke downward, exerting moderate pressure and moving the muscles as they go. When the thumbs reach the top of the spine, the hands are returned to position by a light stroke and the movement is repeated. This is done eight times, with the pressure increased slightly at every repetition until by the fifth time the masseur is bearing down with almost maximum force.

2. Place the fingertips of the right hand at the point where the left trapezius meets the shoulder. Pressing down on the knuckles, with the left hand knead the area in small

clockwise circles, increasing the pressure in the last half of the circle. Knead to the part of the body known as the acromion process (see chart), return the fingers to the original position with a light stroke and begin again. After doing this movement three times, move to the right trapezius and repeat the movement, this time moving in counter-clockwise direction.

3. Place the palms at the tops of the trapezius muscles and stroke down, following the muscles to the shoulders, subtly lessening the pressure as you go. This movement is good for reinforcing the effects of the other two. It should be done from six to ten times.

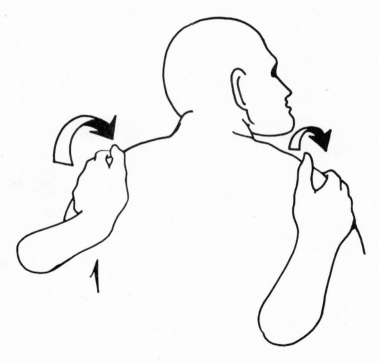

SHOULDERS

The shoulders are usually treated in conjunction with another movement, directed at either neck, back or arms. The only movement devoted purely to the shoulders is the following:

The recipient lies prone, with the masseur taking a position slightly above the middle back. One hand grasps each shoulder. The shoulders are raised together while head and chest remain touching the table. They are rotated in a wide circular pattern, as wide as the recipient can tolerate. Begin the rotation moving from the rear of the body to the front. After six repetitions change direction, moving from the front to the rear. Exert pressure downward to the spine. Cracking noises will accompany this maneuver. They are the sounds of the bones stretching in unfamiliar ways and are totally harmless. Continue this movement until the cracking stops and the shoulders have become easier to maneuver. If the recipient reports pain or discomfort at any time, the movement must be stopped immediately.

After the rotation, stroke the entire shoulder area from the base of the neck and the collarbone right down to the deltoids at the tops of the arms, exerting as much pressure as the recipient can stand. If the muscles are loose enough, petrissage and then tapotement can be performed to good use. If, however, the muscles remain rigid and tense under your fingers, don't try to soften them up with these techniques, but lighten the pressure of your stroking. Sometimes it may be necessary to relax the head and neck before proceeding to the shoulders.

ARMS

The limbs contain islands of different muscles connected by tissue and nerve. Because of the interplay of muscles in the limbs, it is sometimes hard to trace the origin of an ache. It is also impossible to relax a limb just by massaging one part of it. The whole area must be treated.

There are many massage techniques for the arm. You will find that each recipient responds better to some than others, depending upon a particular physical need. Learn as many of the basic techniques as you can, so you can try them out once before pinpointing the ones that are the most effective.

A simple conditioning and relaxing movement for the

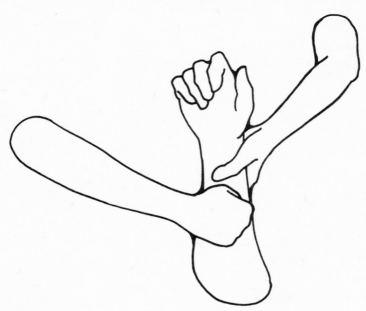

arms is performed by grasping the recipient's wrist between the thumbs and forefingers of both hands, turning the hands in opposite directions and moving up the recipient's arm to the shoulder, exerting enough pressure to push down the skin. When you reach the shoulder, continue down the arm to the wrist with the same movement, lightening the pressure a bit. A more vigorous variation of this movement is done by holding the recipient's wrist firmly with both hands—one on top of the other—and going up and down the arm, lightening the pressure to change position.

Petrissage can be done on the biceps and triceps, the muscles of the front and back, known as the extensor carpi and the flexor carpi. Tapotement is also effective on these muscles, but only if they are sufficiently relaxed.

General deep stroking can be done with the palms or fingers. Stroke up the front and back parts of the arm, keeping the pressure upward, even when returning from shoulder to wrist.

Put your thumb in your armpit and slide it down the back of your arm. You will feel a fairly prominent vein. This is the brachial vein. Move down toward the elbow, using the circular vibrating technique with your thumb or the index and middle fingers of your hand and following the path of this vein. At the elbow switch to the cephalic vein and continue on down to the wrist. These are both sturdy veins and can stand a good bit of pressure.

Flex the arm at the elbow, keeping one hand firmly in the elbow pit and the other at the wrist and exerting pressure on parts of the cephalic vein at these two locations.

Again using the thumb, massage the area around the

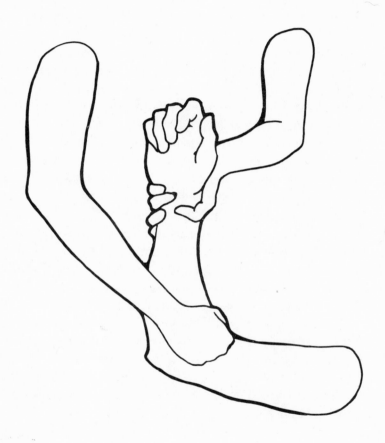

elbow with the circular vibrating technique, exerting maximum comfortable pressure. Lighten pressure when you reach the elbow pit, heighten it again to travel up the arm, passing the bicep, to the armpit. Massage in the armpit, lightening the pressure, and travel down the arm again.

Stroke around the armpit and adjacent areas—the ribcage, pectorals on the upper chest and latissimus dorsi on the back. Petrissage can also be performed on the pectorals and latissimus dorsi after sufficient stroking. Do not use the judo chop technique in this area, even if you're working on a weightlifter with bulging muscles.

On an especially tense person it is sometimes good to massage the hands, relaxing them in preparation for continuing up the arm. The hands and fingers are extremely sensitive to massage.

Hold the recipient's hand palm up in your weaker hand, be it left or right. Using your thumb, massage the muscles of the palm and thumb with the circular vibrating technique. Move up and down the fingers, deep stroking the joints and then, with a light stroke, move to the wrist. Put the recipient's pinky on your palm with the knuckle downward. Massage the joints with your thumb in the circular vibrating technique and work on the cushion or the tip of the finger with the same movement. When you've done this with all the fingers, sandwich the fingers between your palms and, pressing firmly from both sides, stroke with large circular motions.

Now massage the back of the hand, holding the palm loosely and working your thumb from the wrist toward the fingers with small circular movements. Keep the pressure directed toward the wrist. Massage the joints and the knuckles, pulling them out and exerting firm pressure. Move right up to the fingernails.

The important thing about hand and finger massage is thoroughness. Don't begin on one hand, do several fingers and move up to the arm. This type of treatment is taxing on the masseur because it demands patience and great exertion from the thumb and fingers, which are not used to such physical challenges. But once begun it must be seen through to the finish. The hand and all five fingers must be treated before the arm can be massaged.

The individual muscle groups of the arm can be stroked in the following manner:

Both hands grasp the muscle. One hand holds while the other strokes. The thumb of each hand should press on the midline of the muscle, front and back. Stroking is alternate. Pressure is directed downward to the wrist. The hands return to their original positions with light stroking movements.

To stroke the triceps, grasp the lower forearm, raise it slightly to tense the muscle and stroke firmly up to the shoulder, the thumb passing through the midpoint of the muscle, the other fingers moving up along the back of the arm. Return to the original position with a light stroke and repeat the movement until the muscle seems relaxed. Then, as I mentioned earlier, you can continue with petrissage or tapotement.

Kneading is very good for overexerted muscles. To knead the biceps, the arm is raised slightly with one hand supporting the elbow. The thumb is placed in the middle of the flexed muscle, and the other fingers take a firm grip on the side of the arm. Kneading is performed slowly: the hand strokes over the muscles as the position changes.

Move from the beginning of the biceps over the elbow up to the shoulder. Stroke down to the beginning position and repeat the movement.

The narrow muscles of the forearm can also be kneaded in the same manner. Flex the elbow slightly and hold the recipient's hand just above the wrist. Trace a kneading path along the muscles with the thumb. As you change position, your palm will gently stroke the kneaded area. Proceed up to the elbow pit, then stroke back to the original position and begin again. The forearm has two major muscle groups—the medial and lateral. The medial travels right up the middle; the lateral lines the side. With the elbow flexed you can locate these muscles for kneading. Stroking can be done with palms or fingers the way it is done on the rest of the arm.

To perform a thorough arm massage, this is the pattern you must follow:

1. Massage hands and fingers, kneading each muscle and joint and then deep stroking the hands to reinforce the effect.

2. Massage the muscles of the forearm. This can be done quickly unless a special discomfort is located in this area.

3. Massage the elbow and elbow pit, working the joints and muscles until you can feel the relaxation beneath your fingers.

4. Work up the arm, through the biceps, triceps and deltoids, to the shoulder. Concentrate on whatever muscle is particularly tense or weary.

5. Massage the shoulders. Begin by stroking them lightly. If they do not respond to more vigorous movements and the recipient reports discomfort, massage

the neck and the trapezius muscles before returning to them.

Always begin and end an arm massage with light finger stroking in the circular vibrating movement. The slight pressure that is applied should be exerted down toward the wrist. Stroke the inner and outer arm, moving along the pectorals on the chest and the areas on the back directly adjacent to the arms.

BACK

The back is the pivotal area of the human anatomy. Look at the way the body operates and you'll see why. The back is the fulcrum point for the leg and arm muscles. It provides a base for the movements of the head and neck. It lends strength to the other limbs and can sustain a heavier load or more physical exertion over a longer period of time than any other part. The spine is the principal part of the back and of the human skeleton. Some masseurs believe that treatment of the spine can resolve any muscular difficulty anywhere in the body.

Along with this great strength goes great vulnerability. Back ailments are extremely painful and difficult to cure. The slightest twist or strain can cause back pain, making the onset of back trouble very difficult to prevent. People who grew quickly during one point in their childhoods, sometimes develop bad posture, which can lead, in later years, to spinal difficulties. Athletes, accustomed to mighty physical exertion, may get spasms from the slightest movements. Some people who are deskbound for hours at a time have been known to rise from their desks at the end of the day and with the first move they make, whether it be a large stretch or a small reach, double over.

For most people the back is the most sensitive and responsive area to massage. A "back rub" consisting of nothing more than friction applied haphazardly to the back will bring about physical and psychological relaxation. The more sophisticated techniques of back massage can be even more effective.

When massaging the back, take a position on the recipient's left side, standing slightly above the buttocks near the coccyx. Place a pillow under the recipient's abdomen and another one under the ankles if the massage is being given on a table or other hard surface. To present the back in its most natural state the recipient's arms must be down at the sides. Any other position will cause a slight flexing of the back muscles and will impede their relaxation. The head may be turned to either side, but should not be raised above the body. The recipient should not contort his head to see what is going on. Feeling should be more than enough. The recipient should not rest his head on his chin to watch television while being massaged. He should keep it down, resting on one cheek or another.

To condition the muscles of the back and strengthen the spine, perform the following series of massage movements:

1. Place both hands, palms flat, slightly above the buttocks on either side of the spinal column. Pressing down with the heels of the hands, make large circular movements from the small of the back to the shoulders. Exert as much pressure as the recipient can bear and direct it up toward the base of the neck. Cover the whole back, keeping the hands at approximately the same distance

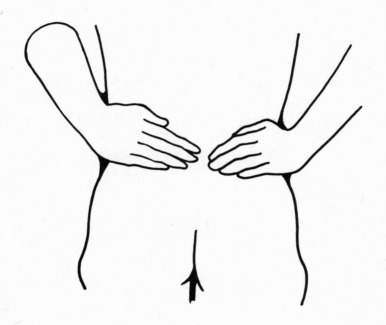

apart. You can repeat this movement as often as the recipient wishes. Three times usually suffices, but this movement has such an immediate relaxing effect that the recipient is loath to have it discontinued.

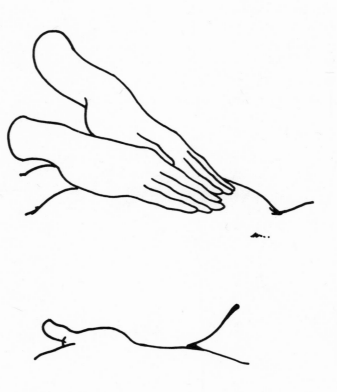

2. Next, trace the spinal vertebrae up the middle of the back until you reach the top one just below the base of the neck. For those who are hungry for technical information, this is called the spinous process of the seventh cervical

vertebra. Place either the thumb or the index and middle fingers on this vertebra and work your way down the vertebrae in small circular strokes until you've reached the coccyx. Massage both knoblike structures of the coccyx and then move up the vertebrae, stopping at the original position. This movement can be repeated with a slight variation. On the way down apply pressure to the right side of the column, instead of directly on top of the vertebrae. When you work your way up do the same, and then for the third and last time, apply pressure on the left side of the column to equalize the effect.

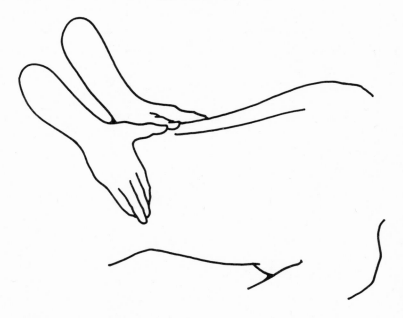

Now knead the muscles on either side of the spinal column. Place the thumb and index fingers of both hands slightly to one side of the spinous process, with the fingers of the left hand above the fingers of the right. Knead the muscle by moving it upward with the left hand and downward with the right, and then reversing the directions. Do this all the way down the back to the sacrum, changing positions with a light stroke. Then move up to a position on the other side of the spinal column and perform the same movements. One treatment on each side should be enough.

Repeat the deep stroking of the back that began the massage, but this time use the whole hand, the fingers stretched out as far as they can go. The circles should be wide, at least nine inches in diameter, and in addition to intense downward pressure, there should be sufficient friction in the rubbing to produce a feeling of warmth on the surface of the skin. Direct pressure up or down toward the heart, depending upon the position of the hands.

Petrissage can then be done on the deltoids, the lower trapezius, the latissimus dorsi and the obliquus externus abdominus. And following the standard pattern, tapotement can be used on the ribcage and the posterior sheet. If cupped-hand tapotement is to be used, the treatment can be extended to the general area of the back. But do not use the judo chop technique on the spinal vertebrae.

If either petrissage or tapotement is done on the back, end the massage by repeating the whole-hand deep stroking movement. This will consolidate the gains of those two movements, smoothing out the treated muscles and restoring the tiny displaced tissues to their proper positions. Pressure should be firm, but not as heavy as it was when the movement was first performed.

Deep stroking and friction are very effective on the whole back and can be begun from a variety of positions.

Digital stroking works well on the smaller muscles and structures of the back, like the spinal vertebrae. It can also be applied with great benefit to the trapezius muscles. Place the thumbs on the outer borders of the trapezii, adjacent to the spinous process. Stroke firmly to the acromia, lifting the muscles away from the skin as you approach the lower cervical region. Return the hands to the original position with a light stroke and perform the movement two or three more times.

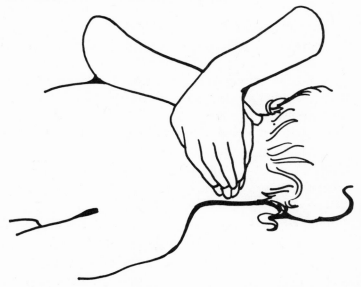

The trapezius muscles also respond well to kneading. Place the fingers of the right hand at the upper cervical regions of the trapezius muscles. Reinforce them with the fingers of the left hand to guarantee firm, controlled pressure. Knead the muscles with firm circular movements to the acromion process and return with a light stroke to the original position.

The muscles of the lower back, so crucial to spinal alignment and muscular flexibility, also respond well to kneading. Place your thumbs on the upper border of the sacrum and knead in small circles—exerting firm pressure upward toward the heart—to the lower border of that muscle. Stroke back to the original position and perform the movement two or three more times. This movement, in conjunction with general back massage, can bring relief from sciatic leg and lower back pain.

If your primary aim is to relax the back, then apply the following sequence of movements:

1. Place the palms on the trapezius muscles with the thumbs resting on the spine. Knead the area around the spine with the thumbs, using moderate to firm pressure directed in toward the spine. Keep the hands on the trapezius muscles and move the thumbs up the neck as far as they will go without forcing the hands to change position. Then move down the neck, retracing your path, using the same small circular movements, and see how far down the spine you can travel before forcing a change of position.

2. Place the hands on the upper back, on either side of the spinal column. Apply stroking-rubbing pressure with the heels of the hands, moving in six-inch circles to the shoulder blades and then back down again. Pressure should be as heavy as possible and should be directed downward toward the coccyx. Move a few inches down from your original position and stroke-rub up to the shoulder blades, returning again. Do this until the entire back has been massaged.

3. Now do this exercise using the three middle fingers

of both hands, with the thumbs resting on the spine. The effect produced is similar to kneading. Lean forward and down on the back until the thumbs are supporting your weight. Perform this exercise until the entire back has been treated.

4. Place the palms on both shoulders, with the heels slightly below. Apply heavy pressure with the palms and stroke with the heels. This is particularly demanding and should not be continued for more than thirty seconds without a few seconds' rest. After the rest, resume pressure and stroking until the movement has been done from three to five times, depending upon the recipient's reaction. Do not repeat this movement more than five times, even if the recipient requests it. You can go back to it in a few minutes or after other techniques have been applied. In general, it is never wise to overdo movements where maximum pressure is exerted.

5. Now place both hands on the upper back, palms flat, thumbs resting about an inch away from either side of the spine. Lean forward and down on the palms until they are supporting your entire weight. Inscribe small, stroking circles with the thumbs while this pressure is being applied, moving down the lateral borders of the spine to the coccyx and then back up to the shoulder blades. This movement is done very slowly and should not be repeated more than once.

6. If the back is adequately relaxed, petrissage can be performed on the deltoids, lower trapezius, latissimus dorsi and obliquus externus abdominis. Following this, tapotement can be employed on the ribcage and the posterior sheet, or extended to the whole back if the

cupped-hand technique is used.

The necessary culmination of this process is a deep stroking movement that begins at the top of the buttocks, on either side of the base of the spine. The heel of the hand is on the buttocks; the palms rest on the small of the back. Applying moderate whole-hand pressure, move up the back in six-inch circles, directing the pressure upward to the heart. When the shoulder blades are reached, stroke down to the original position and spread the hands out a little farther to cover the outer regions of the back. Do this until the entire back has been treated. This movement can be repeated as often as recipient and masseur wish. It will only reinforce the relaxing effects of the other movements.

The two types of back massage I have described here can be used under normal circumstances, after a bath, a sedentary day or a day of exertion. They can also be performed if the recipient complains of tension or muscle aches in the lower back or middle back. DO NOT massage a person who is immobilized by lower back pain or who has a history of recurring lower back ailments. The treatment of such people should be left to orthopedic surgeons and physical therapists. A massage will relieve sciatic or muscular pain; it will ease tension and condition the back. But it cannot cure structural conditions like a slipped disc or sacroiliac problems.

BUTTOCKS

The area of the buttocks can be treated as a prelude to the massage of either the legs or the back. This area includes the buttocks themselves; the coccyx, located just below the spine and above the cleft in the buttocks; and the back part of the hips, found just below the buttocks. Massage of the gluteus medius on the upper part of the buttock can have some effect on the conditioning and relaxation of the lower back; massage of the gluteus maximus can help in the treatment of the legs.

The techniques involved are very simple. Occasionally, tension and pressure are manifested in the coccyx. The recipient reports tightness and/or pain in that area. Simple fingertip stroking of the coccyx is sometimes all that is needed to dispel this pressure. If something more is needed, place the palms flat on the buttocks, the thumbs coming together just above the coccyx. Knead the muscle with firm circular strokes and upward pressure, moving up the back until the palms reach the area occupied by the thumbs at the beginning of the movement. Then move down to the original position. Repeat this movement once or twice.

Another technique for relaxation of the coccyx is begun by grasping the buttocks firmly and placing the thumbs on either side of the coccyx, just below the cleft. Knead the buttocks in an upward direction with the palms while performing circular stroking with the thumbs. Move up the coccyx, stopping at the small of the back and continuing down again to the original position. Repeat this movement two or three times.

The muscles of the buttocks (gluteus maximus and gluteus medius) are kneaded in two fashions. In one, the hands grasp the muscle at its origin and culmination. The muscle is lifted from the skin, and pressure is applied in an upward direction. The palms knead the muscle in alternate movements. Then the other buttock is treated in the same manner.

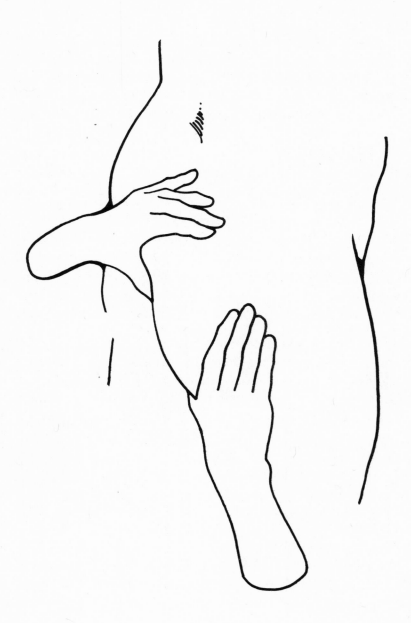

For a deeper kneading effect, grasp the muscle with the right hand supported by the left. Knead the muscle over the colon, using the left hand to provide extra pressure. Perform this same movement on the left buttock as well.

LEGS

Like the back, the legs can become fatigued through immobility as well as exertion. People who sit for hours at a time without once shifting the position of their legs, sometimes rise to discover cramps and stiffness so severe that they impede free movement. The muscles of the legs must endure contortion over long periods of time, especially in this sedentary age when a person will sit hours at a desk and then, after a brief period of stretching and exercise, will return to sit hours more in front of the television.

People who stand on their feet for long periods complain of nonspecific fatigue, which, whether they know it or not, originates in their legs and can be removed by massage. Hindrance of blood circulation is a particular cause of leg pain which can be remedied by massage. Muscle cramps and spasms disappear with astonishing quickness when treated by massage, as do aches in feet.

Most leg massages should begin with general light stroking. The recipient is supine with his arms flexed to the shoulders to avoid interference with the masseur's movements. Reach around the thigh and grasp it with both hands, encompassing as much area as possible. Stroke down to a point just below the knee. Lift the hands in the air and return to the original position. Do this movement four times, then stroke downward from the knee to the ankle in the same manner, returning to the original position and then repeating the movement four times.

Now the leg is ready for more intense conditioning. Grasp the upper thigh with the left hand and place the index and middle fingers of the right hand on the inner side of the leg below the groin. Use the circular vibrating technique to treat the groin area from buttock to hip. Exert moderate to heavy pressure in the direction of the upper groin. Do this on both legs, changing the position of the hands for easier access.

The femoral vein is found in the same general area you have just finished massaging. Follow a circular vibrating path down this vein to the great saphenous vein and from there down to the ankle. Keep the pressure firm and directed up toward the groin.

Lift the muscles of the calves, thighs and buttocks away from the flesh and perform vigorous petrissage. Then judo chop the same areas, taking care to keep the force of your blows firm but bearable.

Grasp the back of the knee with the left hand and apply your thumb to the kneecap, massaging it with circular vibrating motions. Then, increasing the pressure, move the three fingers up the saphenous and femoral veins to the juncture of the groin and the leg.

Now, to reinforce the previous motions, grasp the ankle with one hand and massage the leg from ankle to hip, using four fingers in the circular vibrating technique and then returning to the original position to perform deep palmar strokes along the same path. Massage both sides of the leg, lifting it slightly to get to the back parts. Lighten the pressure with every repetition of the movement.

The long leg muscles respond well to intense palmar

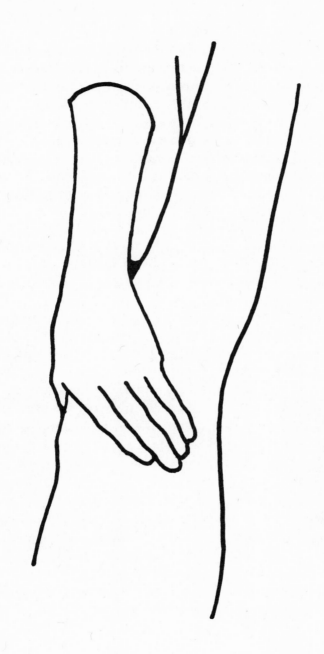

kneading. Because of the sturdiness of the muscles and the great pressure they are subjected to, they sometimes must be exposed to the force and intensity of the kneading process.

The quadricep muscles along the upper leg are kneaded by placing both hands on either side of the kneecap, the left above the right, grasping the muscle between the thumb and forefinger of the left hand, and lifting it away from the skin while the right hand pushes the tissues up toward the hips. Progress up the leg in this manner, stroking to change position. As you approach the origin of the quadriceps, release the left hand and squeeze the muscle with the right all the way up to the groin. Stroke down to the original position and repeat this movement two or three times.

This is the first step in a three-stage kneading process that can be executed on weary or aching legs that have not responded to lighter stroking treatment. The second stage is begun around the rear or posterior surface of the thigh. The knee is flexed slightly to permit access to this area. The right hand takes a position slightly above the knee, the left hand slightly above the right, firmly grasping the muscle of the lower thigh. The same type of kneading movement described above is then performed. Keep the hands close together and the position changes slight. When the left hand reaches the top of the thigh muscle just below the buttock, cross it over the right and back to the muscles of the upper knee. Squeeze the remaining area of muscle with the right hand, and when it reaches the top, stroke lightly down the middle of the thigh until it is resting below the left hand. Recommence the movement, repeating it once or twice, depending upon the reaction of the recipient.

Now, with both hands, grasp the upper area of the thigh, with the thumbs facing each other. Knead down to the top of the knee, the hands alternately rolling the muscle between the palms while the thumbs keep up a steady pressure on the front part of the muscle. When you reach the top of the knee, stroke back to the starting position and repeat this movement two or three times. Complete the series by taking the same position, but deep stroke instead of knead up the top of the thigh, sliding down with the fingertips to the original position and stroking three or four more times.

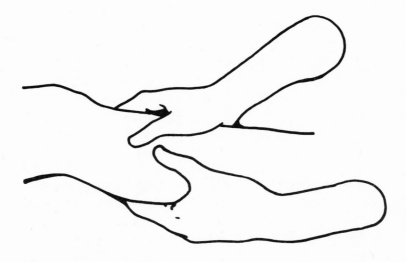

The muscles below the knee can also be kneaded with similar movements. They are a good deal more sensitive than the thigh muscles and must be handled more gently. Begin this process by palm stroking from the knee joint to the ankle joint several times. Put a pillow or rolled-up towel under the knee to give slight elevation without flexing. Place the right thumb over the tibialis anterior and the left thumb as close to it as possible without actually touching. The fingers of the hands grasp the underlying muscle and meet at the medial point. Knead in small circles with the thumbs, exerting pressure upward and outward. As each kneading movement is completed, lightly stroke with the fingers to the next position, repositioning the thumbs and kneading again. Move down to the ankle joint and return to the original position by releasing the fingers and deep stroking upward with the thumbs. Do not perform this movement more than twice.

For the next movement, flex the knee just enough to permit the right hand to slide under it and grasp the knee pit. Place the left palm on the calf muscle slightly below the knee. Knead down toward the ankle with the left hand while the right hand exerts pressure on the knee pit. The muscle should be pulled down away from the knee toward the ankle in the process. At the ankle take a deep palmar stroke to the point of origin and repeat the movement twice. You can then change hands, supporting the knee with the left and kneading with the right to cover another area of the muscle, repeating this movement three times.

Now close the palms over the knee muscles and knead down to the ankle, alternately rolling the muscles between the palms, exerting firm, upward pressure while you move downward. Return to the original position with a deep stroke and repeat this movement twice.

Next, place the heels of the hands at the lower border of the patella, below the kneecap, with the fingers lightly touching the skin above the knee. Execute circular palmar

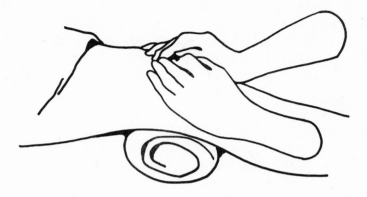

strokes around the knee, with the fingertips just grazing the skin as the heels and palms move. Move up the kneecap slowly in these strokes, and when the heels are above it, return them with a light stroke to the point of origin. Repeat this movement three times.

Place the fingers of both hands around the ankles and stroke upward in circular vibrating motions, exerting firm pressure directed downward. Continue to a point slightly above the kneecap, stroke down to the original position and repeat this movement three times.

By now you're probably familiar with the last movement in the massage of an entire part of the anatomy. It is the deep palmar stroke, intended to readjust displaced tissue, soothe newly conditioned muscle and relieve the strain caused by some of the more intense movements. Completing the kneading process of the leg is even more important than completing the circular vibrating treatment. The movements have been more forceful, contact with the muscle has been more intimate, and more

71

actual manipulation of tissue has taken place. So, after the digital stroking of the lower leg has been executed, close the palms around the ankles and move upward in one uninterrupted stroke to the top of the thighs, sliding down with fingertips or nails to the original position and repeating the movement as many times as the recipient is willing and the masseur is able. The recipient can go from a supine to prone position to give better access to the backs of the legs during the course of the massage. This, however, is not necessary, and the constant changing of positions might diminish the effect of the massage.

FEET

There is no pill you can take for aching or cramped feet. The only effective treatment is one that is directed at the ailing muscles themselves—baths, local medications and especially massage.

The masseur prepares the foot for massage by light stroking from the ankle to the tips of the toes. The sole of the foot is cushioned in the palm of the right hand while the fingers of the left stroke down with firm pressure. Begin at the anklebone and follow a straight path over the instep to the toes and on either side of the instep. Cover the whole foot twice before going on to another movement.

The second step in a foot massage is the thumb kneading of the dorsum of the foot (see diagram). Grasp the sole of the foot with the palms and place the thumbs under the anklebone on the right side. Knead in small circular movements over the ankle to the metatarsal joints on the other side of the foot, then stroke back with the thumbs to the original position, replacing the hands when you are ready to begin again. Press firmly, rolling the muscles underneath your thumbs, and repeat the movement once.

Now place the thumbs at the base of the toes, the right thumb under the big toe, the left one under the little toe, edging toward the outer border of the sole. Stroke laterally across the foot, the thumbs going in opposite directions. Do this by keeping the thumbs and hands still and pushing the elbows out from the chest and back again, forcing their movement. Pressure should be firm and directed along the path of the stroke. When you reach the heel, stroke lightly up to the original position and begin again, repeating this

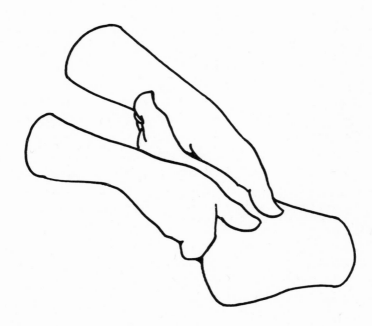

movement once or twice, depending upon the reaction of the recipient.

Next, grasp the toes with the left hand, cup the right hand slightly and place the side used for judo chops at the base of the toes. Exerting deep pressure, stroke down the sole toward the heel, turning the hand so that it ends the movement with the palm flat on the table. Lift your hand and re-establish the position, repeating this movement three times.

Put the hands together with the thumbs crossed. Place the fingers at the base of the toes on the front part of the foot. Stroke up toward the ankle, exerting deep pressure. When you reach the ankle, let the fingers of the right hand stroke over to the right side of the anklebone in several circular vibrating strokes, while the fingers of the left do the same on the left side of the ankle. Keep the thumbs crossed and pressing down on the instep. Stroke lightly back to the point of origin and repeat the movement three times.

Lift the foot slightly and grasp the ankle with the left hand. Place the palm of the right hand at the heel and deep stroke up over the toes to the instep and up to the ankle in one movement. Slide back to the original position and cover the whole foot, stroking up the sole and diverging to the right, the left and then back up the medial point of the instep. Most masseurs complete a foot massage by putting the foot back down on the table and deep stroking with the palms up the leg to the thigh. If you have already completed a leg massage, this is a superfluous movement, but if you plan to continue with one, it is a good way to reinforce the foot massage and prepare for the movements to come.

Some people are extremely ticklish on the soles of the feet and between the toes. If stroked too lightly in these areas they ·withdraw their feet. But firm pressure on these areas usually alleviates this ticklishness and permits the massage to continue.

CHEST

There are several simple techniques for the massage of the chest. They should be done quickly as a component in the whole-body massage process. Conditioning and relaxation of the chest muscles is not as crucial as it is in other parts of the body.

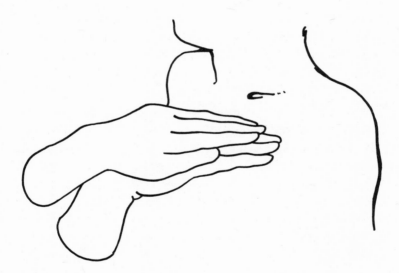

Place the fingers of each hand at the point where the clavicle meets the sternum. Use the circular vibrating technique to stroke to the ends of the clavicle. Keep the pressure as deep as possible and directed down toward the heart. Stroke back to the original position and move the fingers down a bit to a position below the clavicle. Again stroke out until you reach the shoulders or, as you continue down the sternum, the latissimus dorsi. If the recipient is a woman, do not massage the sensitive areas of the breast, but restrict yourself to the less delicate upper areas. If the recipient is a male, move all the way down the sternum to the ribcage, lightening the pressure as you execute circular vibrating movements in this area. Stroke back to the original position and execute this movement two or three more times.

Then place the heels of the hands below the ribcage on either side of the sternum and stroke up in three-inch circles to the shoulders. Again, avoid the protuberant parts of the female breast. Stroke down with the palms to the original position and perform this movement twice more.

Now perform petrissage on the pectoral, vigorously squeezing out that length of muscle between the shoulders and the breast, and again avoiding the sensitive areas of the female breast. Stroke back to the point of origin with the fingers and repeat the movement once. If your pressure has been heavy enough, the recipient will not request another repetition.

Follow this with a judo chop attack to the ribcage, moving up and down the length of the sternum in the male, avoiding the breasts in the female. Remember, the force of your blows cannot be as heavy as on the back, legs or abdomen. Keep them brisk and firm, but do not give yourself the liberty of bearing down the way you may have done on the other parts.

Stroke the entire chest area again, this time with the middle fingers of the hands in circular vibrating movements. Complete the massage by repeating the vigorous heel-stroke movement.

ABDOMEN

In the abdominal massage the masseur stands on the recipient's right side over the knees so that the hands must reach slightly to get to the massaged area. The recipient is lying supine. The knees are flexed slightly and supported with a pillow.

Begin all abdominal massages with a superficial stroking of the entire area. Place the hands over the lower borders of the ribcage, the thumbs meeting at the bottom of the sternum. Stroke lightly in three-inch circles down to the top of the pubic area, known as the symphysis pubis. Lift the hands, re-establish the position and repeat the movement three more times until the recipient reports a feeling of relaxation in the abdomen.

Next, place the fingertips of both hands at the symphysis pubis, with the thumbs almost touching under the navel. Make deep circular strokes around this area toward the spine. Trace the crest of the ilium around to the back until the fingers meet at the upper lumbar vertebrae. Then stroke forward with the palms to the waistline. Lift hands, re-establish position and repeat the movement three times. Keep the pressure firm, but remember, the purpose of abdominal massage is to treat the muscles of the abdomen, not to exert pressure on the

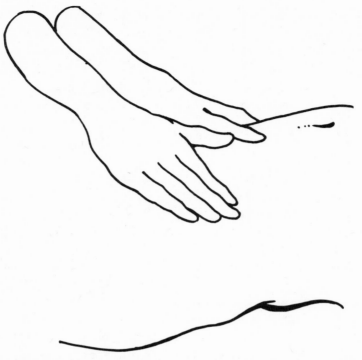

visceral organs. In positions where the abdomen is not
flexed and its muscles are not brought into prominence,
don't exert maximum pressure.

After you have deep stroked the lower abdomen, you
can repeat essentially the same movement on the upper
regions. Place the right palm at the base of the sternum so
that the fingers lie over the inner border of the left ribs.
With the left hand over the right for reinforcement, stroke
lightly across the ribs and down over the upper abdominal
muscles, returning to the point of origin with a firm stroke
over the upper abdominal muscles. Repeat this movement
four times, then reverse positions so that the palm is now

over the inner border of the right ribs. Stroke down and over in the same manner, returning to the original position with a firm stroke over the upper abdomen and repeating this movement three times.

The colon is now kneaded in the following manner:

Cup the right hand and place it over the lower right part of the abdomen, beneath the navel, so that only the judo chop side of the hand is in contact with the skin. Grasp the right wrist with the left hand for reinforcement. Press down slightly and shovel up the muscles, rolling the hand over the abdomen and closing the fingertips in toward the palm. When the right hand has almost been closed into a fist, move the fingertips to a point slightly to the right of the area just massaged, return the hand to its original position and begin the shoveling movements again. Perform this movement all the way across the colon, re-establishing position with a firm fingertip stroke over the lower abdomen and across to the point of origin. Repeat this movement twice. Now, using the fingers of the right hand, reinforced by the fingers of the left, deep stroke the same area you have just kneaded, moving upward over the ascending colon and downward over the descending colon. Stroke lightly back to the point of origin and repeat the movement five times.

Grasp the tissues on the right side of the abdomen between the palms. Keep the hands motionless and produce kneading movements by pulling the elbows out from the sides and returning them. Progress across the abdomen in this manner, returning to the point of origin with a light palmar stroke. Repeat this movement three times.

Now conclude this massage by deep stroking the entire

abdominal area with the palms, beginning with deep pressure and slowly lightening it until you complete the movement by barely skimming the skin with the fingertips.

That is only one of the many ways to massage the abdomen. Athletes who are primarily concerned with conditioning the muscles of the abdomen for strength and endurance can make use of another combination of movements.

First, lightly stroke the area with the fingertips, slowly increasing pressure until after three or four movements it is quite heavy. Then place a pillow or rolled-up towel under the feet, causing the abdominal muscles to flex slightly. Place the heels of the hand on the symphysis pubis and stroke in heavy three-inch circles along the muscle.

Now raise the elevation under the feet to bring the muscle into greater prominence. Perform petrissage on the entire abdominal region.

Now have the recipient raise his legs six inches in the air, so that the muscles visibly protrude. Execute the judo chop technique, beginning with a steady rain of blows from a height of several inches and increasing the height and force of the blows until the recipient reports discomfort. This technique can be repeated until the recipient can easily bear the hardest and highest blows you can inflict.

With the heels of the hands, stroke the area around the hips, moving up along the sides of the torso to the armpits and then back down again. Avoid the abdominal muscles—they will be relaxing from the strain of the tapotement—and keep the pressure heavy and directed upward, even when moving back down toward the hips.

Consolidate the effects of the massage by stroking in

circular vibrating movements around the entire abdominal area, slowly lightening the pressure until it is a feather-like touch. Remove one hand and stroke the area with the fingertips or fingernails of the other. Conclude by tracing a grazing circle around the navel, light enough to induce shivers in the recipient.

I have just described in detail some of the techniques used to condition and relax the major muscles of the body.

Instructions for the various massage movements are explicit and must be followed to the letter. There are other techniques that I have not covered, all of which have been developed over the years by physicians, physical therapists and others who are concerned with the conditioning and maintenance of the human body. You cannot create your own movements. And don't think you can! The body is constructed in a certain way, and only certain types of manipulation will be beneficial to it. Of course, you can lightly stroke in any area and direction you wish; the effects are minimal and harmless. But in movements where pressure and manipulation are involved, stick closely to the described techniques, or you might find yourself doing a lot of unintentional harm to the recipient.

CHAPTER VII

VARIATIONS

Certain national groups have made a specialty of massage. The Swedes and the Japanese, for instance, seem especially preoccupied with the proper care and exercise of the body. They have ritualized the bath-massage procedure, making it an integral part of their culture. Most of the techniques I described in the last chapter are components of Swedish massage. They are performed in combination with other movements, as well as steam treatments, baths and the use of various striking implements—willow branches, palm leaves, etc. A complete Swedish massage usually lasts at least an hour. At its completion the body should be relaxed but fatigued enough at least from the exertion to send the recipient into a short, restful slumber.

The typical Swedish massage involves concentrated

manipulation of the major parts of the body—the back, legs, arms, neck and abdominal region. Among the techniques used are two distinctly Swedish variations. In the stroking or effleurage movement, the Swedes place pressure and take whiskbroom strokes of six to twelve inches along the surface of the skin, moving always in the direction of the heart. In lieu of the circular vibrating movement, they press the index and middle fingers down hard on the muscle and move them back and forth over it, producing a slightly different sensation more akin to kneading than stroking.

The massage usually takes place after a steam or sauna bath. Most gyms and health clubs are equipped with either or both of these. Portable models of the sauna bath are also available commercially.

North American Sauna of Huntington Station, Long Island, New York, has a variety of home saunas that will fit the need of the careful shopper. I highly recommend their use to you.

I personally feel that the sauna in itself can be a fantastic experience, even if it is not possible for you to have a massage right afterwards. You'll find that the more times you go in and out of the sauna with an ice-cold shower in between, the more freely you'll perspire. Once you get used to taking a sauna bath regularly, that will be the only time you'll feel completely clean from within.

Those who do not have access to a sauna can create one in their own bathrooms. Close the windows and doors, and seal off all the areas in the room through which air might escape. Turn the shower on—the hot water only—and let it run until the room is full of steam. If your shower is in a tub, plug the drain up to keep the water in. If it is in a stall, place a mat or towel over the drain to get some accumulation of water. When the tub or stall is full to overflowing, uncover the drain, letting the water out. Keep the hot water running; whatever it adds to your fuel bill will be worth it. When the tub or stall is almost empty, replug the drain. Do this until the bathroom is enveloped in fog. Stay in the room for as long as you can tolerate the heat and moisture, turning the water on to produce more steam, if necessary. Some people feel that the steam heat makes the body most receptive to massage, and they perform massages in the sauna. Others prefer to see the Swedish bath ritual to the end before having a massage.

The willow branch technique can also be performed in the sauna or later during the massage. The movement involves a gentle striking of the back with a bunch of loosely-held branches. Willow branches are prescribed, and they are the only ones that should be used. Don't try the technique with maple or oak branches; they are not pliant enough and will only cause discomfort. Do not whip with the branches, but strike gently, moving up and down the back, including the back of the legs and arms if the recipient so desires. Do this for from two to ten minutes, depending upon the recipient's tolerance. If the willow branches are used during the sauna, a little time should be allowed between the treatment and the transfer to the next activity.

If all this is taking place in your own bathroom, unseal the room to let some of the hot air escape, and modulate the temperature of the water until it is just right for a very hot, but bearable shower. Get under the shower, soaping and rinsing yourself completely. Now you are ready for a treatment with the palm leaves. This can be self-administered or done by the masseur, depending upon the level of intimacy. The palm leaf has a mildly abrasive edge. Soap yourself again from head to toe and brush the leaf against your body, starting at the back of the neck and working all the way down to your toes. Coming on the heels of the willow branch treatment and the expansion and softening of the skin by the hot shower, the palm leaves impart a tingling sensation even to normally desensitized parts of the body.

Rinse again, this time gradually eliminating the hot water and adding cold until the shower is as icy as you can make it. If you have a needle spray attachment, by all means use it now. The contrast in heat and texture will penetrate to your very bones. Step out of the shower, dry yourself with thick Turkish towels and step over to the bed or the massage table. After a comprehensive whole-body massage followed by a brisk alcohol rub, you probably won't be in the mood for anything else but a good nap. You'll awake refreshed, and you'll be ready for anything.

The Swedes are great believers in contrast, both in temperature and texture. The alternation of soft and hard, caress and rub, hot and cold is the cornerstone of their conditioning techniques. The practice of applying hot and cold towels is another technique developed by the Swedes. It is most frequently used to open and close the pores of men's faces after a shave, but it is also an excellent adjunct to cosmetic-conditioning facial massage for both sexes. Fold a thick, fluffy Turkish towel in quarters and dip it in a pan of near-boiling water. Wring the towel out—you may need rubber gloves—and air it for about thirty seconds, then open it and lay it gently across the subject's face, leaving only the nose uncovered for breathing. Wait a few seconds for the subject to become accustomed to the heat and then mold the towel around the contours of the face. Keep the towel on until most of the heat has gone out of it. Then remove and perform the facial massage movements I described in the last chapter. The equivalent of tapotement for facial massage is light slapping with the fingers around the jowls and cheekbones. Do this after you've completed the massage movements and before a final brisk rubdown of the entire facial area.

After the massage apply another hot towel, but keep this one on for no more than a minute or two. While it is on, take another towel and immerse it in a pan of cold water. No ice or refrigeration is necessary; water from the bathroom tap will run sufficiently cold. Apply the cold towel and keep it on until the cold has gone out of it and it is merely a damp rag. Then dab witch hazel or any sort of bracing cologne around the face and neck. The actual physical effect of this type of treatment is negligible. It is not a facelift and does not actually tone up sagging muscles or wipe out wrinkles. What it does is relieve facial fatigue. When people are exhausted, mentally or physically, they lack the will to adequately support the burden of their bodies. Facial massage brings an incredible infusion of vigor into the muscles. The subject looks younger and healthier, merely because he or she has regained strength and spirit, not because any physiological miracles have been performed.

The hot and cold towel treatment can be applied to other parts of the body that are particularly tense or exhausted. It is effective at the base of the spine or neck.

The Japanese are so convinced of the therapeutic,

erotic, tranquilizing and absolutely curative properties of the bath that they have ritualized the entire bathing process. The bathing facilities in a Japanese home are housed in a special room of their own. The family bath is a daily ritual, and one of the first things that parents and children do after a long absence from one another is hop into the bath.

Because of the communal nature of the Japanese bath, the actual tub is a good deal larger than any found in Europe or America. Unless you want to go to the expense of building one, you'll have to be content with the single or double style of bathing used in the West.

Because bathing is a group activity in Japan, it is considered the height of rudeness to enter a tub with a dirty body. Bathers cleanse themselves thoroughly in a vat of water by the bath, rubbing themselves vigorously with soap and the *tawashi* or Japanese washcloth, a rough-textured abrasive vegetable fabric, and entering only when they have cleansed all the surface dirt from their bodies.

The size of the standard Japanese tub affords a great deal of maneuvering space to the bathers, which means that many variations of massage can be performed in the bath itself.

Real Japanese massage should not be performed by amateurs. It also should not be given to people who have not been warned beforehand about its methods and effects. A brief description of a few standard Japanese massage movements should indicate why I advise caution.

The Japanese believe in conditioning by shock and torsion; hence, the following two movements:

1. The subject sits on the floor, legs crossed and folded

under the haunches. The masseur stands behind, directly over the shoulders. The shoulders are firmly grasped and the torso is turned back and forth quickly and vigorously with pressure exerted down and out. If the masseur does not hear the sharp cracking of bones and vertebrae, the movement is not forceful enough, and efforts must be intensified. This movement can also be performed with the masseur sitting behind the subject, elbows under the subject's armpits and hands clasped behind the subject's neck in what wrestlers call a full-nelson. The neck and spine are more directly manipulated in this position, and the cracks are even more audible.

2. This is the Japanese cure for a stiff neck. It is very effective, if executed correctly. Again, the subject sits with the masseur standing behind, directly over the shoulders. The masseur places one hand on top of the subject's head, the other on the subject's chin, the fingers spreading slightly down the subject's neck. The masseur waits until the subject's body is relaxed—which can only be when a sudden blow is not expected—and then suddenly twists the neck in the direction of the pain or stiffness. Again, the sound of cracking bones and vertebrae must be heard. But even if they are not, this maneuver should not be repeated immediately thereafter.

The next two movements also conform to the Japanese theory of shock and pressure.

1. To cure a headache, the subject lies supine with eyes closed and hands at sides. The masseur places his thumbs on the closed eyelids, the fingers gripping the crown of the head. The thumbs are kept there, gently touching the eyelids, until the subject is sufficiently relaxed, and then the masseur presses downward with firm pressure on the

eyes, squeezing the scalp in the same movement. Working on the principle of extrusion, this is supposed to shoot new blood into the brain. Pressure should be kept up as long as the subject can stand it—which certainly won't be long—and then released. The movement should not be repeated for a little while afterward.

2. Another therapeutic-conditioning movement is performed on the entire front torso region, from abdomen to the lungs. This is illustrative of the marvelous economy of Japanese massage. This one movement affects the stomach, ribs, chest cavity and lungs, and is executed in the space of a few seconds. The subject lies supine, and the masseur places his right hand on the subject's stomach, palm flat, reinforcing it with the stiffened fingers of the left hand. Again there is a pause to give the subject a chance to relax from the tense anticipation of the movement. At the right moment the masseur suddenly presses downward on the stomach. This causes all the air to escape from the lungs, and the entire pulmonary area collapses like an empty bladder. Blood also temporarily flows from the stomach, returning in a warm rush as the air returns to the lungs. This movement can be performed several times. Subject and masseur should be especially careful of the natural resistance offered by the muscles to this sort of harsh, sudden manipulation. Another crucial principle is the total passivity of the subject, the total yielding of physical autonomy to the masseur.

When the Japanese knead, they knead with a vengeance. After a vigorous back massage, with much chopping and wrenching of limbs, the subject takes a prone position on the floor. The masseur then steps lightly on the subject's back, balancing on the toes for several seconds and then coming down with both feet at the base of the spine. Kneading is done by walking up and down the back of the subject, pressing and turning with the balls and heels of the feet. This movement is made a little less frightening by the twenty- to forty-pound difference in weight between the average Japanese and his Western equivalent. Still, having someone walk on your back can feel murderous and should be done by a competent Japanese masseur, not one of your friends who has nothing better to do.

The Japanese also have a movement in which the masseur stands on the subject's stomach and springs lightly up and down on his toes without ever losing contact with the skin. As you might think, this is a terrific conditioner for the abdominal muscles, but should be used only on someone whose abdominal muscles are in pretty good condition to begin with.

There are as many different movements in Japanese massage as there are in any other form. I have just given examples which best illustrate the basic massage philosophy of the Japanese. Shock and pressure for the Japanese; contrasts in temperature, pressure and stroke for the Swedes. Both systems of massage aim to accomplish the same thing, but with vastly different techniques.

CHAPTER VIII

MECHANICAL MASSAGE

Wilhelmina, the famous model who now runs her own agency, says that after a particularly hard day at the office she likes to unwind with a hot bath followed by a complete back rubdown by her TV producer husband, Bruce Cooper. Bruce uses warm oil as lubrication and straps an electric vibrator on each hand.

In the utopian future every home will be equipped with a robot masseur, programmed for all types of massage, gentle, totally selfless and on call twenty-four hours a day. Until that great day comes, we can become gradually more accustomed to automated massage by the variety of massage aids that have been put on the market in the last few years. Unconsciously, we are being weaned away from the one-to-one human massage ratio that has prevailed for centuries. Whether this is good or bad, I don't know. But these machines are efficient, and, as long as the intimacy of human contact is preserved, can be used to great advantage in massage.

VIBRATORS

These are the best-known of the massage aids. Run by electric or battery power, they simulate the effect of stroking or kneading—depending upon how they are used—but with a speed and regularity that no human masseur could possibly duplicate. When used by a trained masseur, there is no doubt that they heighten the penetration of the massage. But the reason for the sudden upsurge in their popularity is the discovery that they can be put to very profitable erotic use.

The most common vibrator in use consists of a three-finger grip under an electric motor. This is used most often by barbers for a quick scalp massage after a haircut. The action of the motor causes the fingers to vibrate slightly as they administer the massage. This type of vibrator was the first to be used in body massage. As a mechanical aid to what remains essentially manual manipulation, it is very effective. I do find, however, that after prolonged use the masseur tends to let the vibrator do the work instead of his fingers. Because this model is made specifically to be used in conjunction with hand and finger movements, this kind of laziness renders it practically useless. When using one of these machines, be aware that your fingers are actually the vibrators and they have to participate somewhat in the entire massage process.

The vibrator that has caused all the furor is the cylindrical type, now sold in most drugstores for five dollars and under. It is usually from four to eight inches long and about an inch in diameter. It consists of a battery-operated motor covered in soft plastic, with or without a rubberized tip. It is held in the hand or loosely in the fingers and passed gently over the area to be massaged. The little motor is quite powerful and can cause quite a sensation. This type of vibrator can be used for whole-body massage, but its effectiveness will be compromised by the smallness of its contact area. It will be almost like performing the circular vibrating technique with one finger instead of three or four; massage time will be lengthened, impatience will result, and because of this less of the body will be massaged than if done in the conventional manual fashion.

Those who are primarily interested in conditioning and relaxation would do better with a pistol-grip vibrator. This is the machine most used by chiropractors and professional masseurs. It is held like a pistol, with the massage head moved over the skin. The more expensive models have interchangeable heads for scalp, facial and body massage. When using a vibrator, follow the paths used in standard manual massage. Keep the pressure a bit lighter; the machine will supply the extra force. There is a tendency to overuse vibrators. Because their application is much less taxing for the masseur than actual manual manipulation, less care is taken in adjusting the pressure and repetition of the movements. You must follow the book exactly, tracing the same paths and making the same number of repetitions, or your results will be negligible.

These vibrators fulfill their promise of providing an effective massage. But there are other types—commonly known as oscillators—for which their proponents make claims that cannot be fulfilled. The oscillator most frequently encountered is a machine with a strap attachment found in health clubs and reducing salons. You are told to place the strap around some flabby area that you wish to trim down and turn on the machine. The vibration of the machine causes the strap to jiggle violently around your body, turning and jostling the flab, but doing nothing to make it disappear. The sensation produced may be pleasant—an illusion of vigor and slimness in the obese parts—but the results are nil. The only way to lose weight and regain trimness is to exercise and to moderate your diet. Massage helps, but it is not a short cut. The oscillator does nothing but shake up your vital organs to no avail.

The other type of oscillator has a steel shaft to which are attached a variety of small rubber tips. An electric motor makes the shaft turn, and the tips simulate the circular vibrating movement.

Not all vibrators are electric-powered. The force of driving water has proved just as effective in producing the type of mechanical movement needed for massage. There is a vibrator that can be attached to the head of the shower and can be used for intensive whole body massage.

This is a rather common type of vibrator that consists of a head equipped with scores of tiny bristles. When the water is turned on, the bristles pulsate at 1,000 times a minute, while a stream of water is also driven through the head. The sensation is as intense as electric vibration, and since this vibrator is used in a shower, the heat and pressure of the water opens the pores and makes the body even more susceptible to the benefits of massage.

My personal preference is the *VibraSpa* Massager which I use in conjunction with VibraSpa's effervescent natural mineral crystal baths. This massager, I have found, permits me for the first time to massage my entire body comfortably in warm water. And because there is no plug and there are no wires I don't have to worry about shocks.

The VibraSpa Massager has a flat surface and a contoured surface that help me dissipate the occasional aches and pains at the end of a busy day. The VibraSpa mineral crystals I use contain ingredients found in the world's most famous spas. In addition, they contain Vitamins A and D.

It has been my practice to use two capfuls of these effervescent crystals in my bath three times a week and my massager. I would urge that the same regimen by any woman will tend to make her feel infinitely better than she did before. And to feel better is to look better, as every woman knows instinctively.

I use the massager's flat surface for back muscles and its contoured surface for arms, shoulders, legs, and feet. I return to the flat surface for that all-important facial.

Every woman is not born with soft and lovely skin. But every woman can do things to make her skin softer and lovelier. This combination of massage and mineral crystals, I think, is a move in that direction of improving one's skin, and, at the same time, bringing true relaxation to the body.

WHIRLPOOLS

The curative, relaxing effects of swiftly moving hot water have been appreciated for centuries. Sprains and strains and various types of tears in the musculature respond very well to this type of treatment. The whirlpool bath is the perfect marriage of heat and movement. Large models which permit total immersion of the body are found in gyms, health clubs and physical therapy centers. The whirling action is usually produced by the injection of compressed air into the water, although in the smaller units the water is agitated in much the same manner as in a washing machine. The swirling movement of the water penetrates a good deal more than you might think, simulating the deep stroking movement of massage. Not only is it good for muscular problems, but it is recommended for disorders of the gastrointestinal and urogenital systems as well.

To be truly therapeutic, the whirlpool must be extremely rapid. Most home models are used in the bathtub, and as yet it has proven impossible to safely produce such rapidity of movement for a relatively small space. But, although a home whirlpool cannot be truly therapeutic, it can be a good prelude to massage.

It is my personal opinion that any individual who chooses to use such a whirlpool should do so very carefully. The home whirlpool in the hands of an unskilled amateur can aggravate an already existing condition.

Another massage aid that has recently come into prominence is the alternating pressure mattress. Once used exclusively in the care of invalids or bedridden patients, this device is now being used by normal people for an extra fillip of massage treatment while they sleep. An inflatable plastic mattress equipped with protruding air tubes, it is placed over a standard mattress and under the bottom sheet. An electrically-powered motor causes the air tubes to inflate and deflate, delivering a gentle massage to the parts of the body in contact. The mattress is totally silent and the device can be safely used while the subject is asleep. For those who choose sleep over massage, it is a good way to relieve soreness and tension in muscles during slumber. Of course its effects do not equal those of massage, but people treated to its gentle manipulations over a period of hours report marked relief.

Vibrator beds have become a staple item in most hotels and motels. You insert a quarter into a coin box to start the machine, and a motor located in the center of the mattress sends a vibrating action, which lasts from fifteen minutes to a half hour, throughout the entire bed. The sensation is quite pleasant, and if you've got a handful of quarters, you can pass a very pleasant evening.

MEDIA

Media is the masseur's term for the types of external lubrication used on the skin during massage. The medium must fulfill three separate functions:

1. Conditioning of the skin.
2. Prevention of chafing and irritation.
3. Heightening of the sensations of the massage, or producing sensations of its own.

If you want to condition as well as lubricate, pick on a cream or oil with therapeutic qualities. Masseurs use a variety of conditioning lubricants made from olive oil, glycerine, coconut oil, oil of sweet almonds, in addition to the traditional lubricants: petroleum jelly, lanolin and cold cream. Cocoa butter is considered especially potent in restoring texture to cracked or stretched skin. Women use it on their nipples after childbirth to keep the skin soft and flexible.

If you are massaging a particularly hirsute male and you want to avoid tangling or twisting the hair on his back, chest or limbs, spread a thin coating of talcum powder or French chalk on the massage surface. Do not use olive or mineral oil, or you will only compound your problem. Powders have the advantage of providing a relatively smooth massage surface without detracting from the all-important "feel" of the skin. Most professionals prefer them over other media for this reason. But they are not conditioners.

Oils and creams are quite acceptable for the hairless parts of the body. I spoke before of the ancients' strong belief in the curative qualities of olive oil. This medium is very good for a face and neck massage, if the subject doesn't mind the smell. It will impart a temporary sheen to the skin, even after being washed off, as will most of the other massage oils.

Cold creams are soothing. When you use them, be careful not to overapply. Use the type that absorbs easily into the skin without leaving an oily residue. Rub in small amounts at a time, until the surface is well lubricated. Then pass a moist towel over the area to remove the excess cream.

Some people like the cool feel of a cream or a lotion against the skin during a massage. Most of the creams and astringent lotions remain cool if kept at room temperature. But if you want to give the subject a pleasant shock, leave the cream or lotion in the refrigerator for about an hour before the massage, taking it out just as you begin.

Most professional massages are concluded with an alcohol rub. As a medium, alcohol has several valuable properties. It closes pores which have been opened wide by heat and manipulation. This protects the body against the absorption of dirt and infection once it ventures out of the sterile confines of the massage room. It also provides needed insulation, an antifreeze for those going from a warm room to a wintry street. In the first moments of its application, alcohol produces a cold, bracing sensation, but as it penetrates through the skin, a feeling of warmth seeps through the body; the treated muscles seem to glow under its influence. If the subject has sustained minor cuts or scratches during the massage, alcohol is a good disinfectant and astringent. And for those who want to exude a clean, pleasant fragrance without recourse to perfumes, it is the perfect choice. Alcohol also helps to remove excess cream or lotion from the skin without the necessity of soap and water.

Never mix your media in a massage. Don't dream up creative combinations of lotions and creams. Don't smear the body with so much lubricant that the hands slide over the surface ineffectually. If you plan to conclude with an alcohol rub, apply your massage creams or lotions sparingly. Don't rub a perfumed lotion or cream onto the body after you have used the alcohol. There is a little bit of the mad scientist in all of us. The urge to tamper with all the tempting bottles and jars leads to a gooky, unmanageable mess on the body. As in everything else, moderation is the key word in using media.

CHAPTER IX

DOING IT YOURSELF

We all endure many moments of tension during a busy day. A sudden headache or muscle spasm is brought on by some unpleasant news. Your neck stiffens from holding your head in one position for too long. You get a cramp in the calf; you make an awkward turn after several hours of immobility, and you suddenly have an annoying ache in your shoulder. With this tightness comes irritability, loss of concentration, insomnia—the symptoms multiply almost endlessly.

Sometimes two aspirins will bring the spiral of pain to a quick end. This cure is not quite as satisfying as a good massage, but it will work occasionally. For muscle aches and the trace pains of psychic tension, a massage treatment has more dimensions to it than any chemical remedy. And if there is no time for a conventional massage, or no masseur readily available, you can give yourself a massage.

There is a ten-minute whole-body massage that you can perform on yourself during coffee breaks, upon rising in the morning or before retiring for the night. It is not as effective as a complete massage administered by another, but it will ameliorate any minor symptoms of physical or mental strain. The self-massage movements can be executed in the following series:

1. Place the thumb of one hand on the wrist of the other, exerting light pressure in the area of the pulse. Using circular vibrating strokes, massage up the front of the arm, directing the pressure up toward the shoulder. When you reach the clavicle, slide down with a deep stroke along the biceps and return to the original position. Repeat this movement once. Then place the thumb on the back of the wrist at the bone and massage up the back of the arm to the top of the deltoid, sliding down to repeat that movement once.

2. Perform petrissage on the arm muscles, grasping them between the thumb and fingers of the hand, squeezing and rolling gently. Begin on the inside of the forearm and move upward to the armpit, returning to the point of origin with a deep palmar stroke, then moving up the other side of the arm over the triceps to the top of the deltoids. Perform these petrissage movements only once.

3. Massage the elbow by placing the thumb in the hollow of the elbow pit and the other fingers around the back of the elbow, on either side of the elbow bone. Press down with the thumb and massage the elbow bone with the circular vibrating technique, exerting as much pressure as you can bear.

4. Grip the palm of the hand with the thumb and two

middle fingers. Knead the palm, beginning at a point just above the wrist and continuing up to the first joints of the fingers. Knead the entire area, working slowly, exerting firm pressure. Now turn to the back of the hand and repeat the kneading process. Cover the entire hand in this manner, working on each of the fingers separately, the kneading thumb moving from back to front. Go over every separate bone and joint in the hand. When you have finished the massage, rub the hand briskly with the palm of the other.

5. Perform the same series of movements on the other hand.

6. Place your two hands along the back of your neck, thumbs at the trapezius muscles, fingers moving up the back of the neck to the hairline. Massage the area with circular vibrating strokes, moving up to the scalp and back down again with a deep stroke. Repeat this movement two or three times.

7. Perform petrissage on the trapezius muscles of the neck and on the sternocleidomastoid muscles.

8. Perform light tapotement on the same area, striking on both sides of the neck with each hand. Make the treatment light and rapid. When you stop, you will be amazed to feel the flow of blood and relaxation in that area.

9. Now massage the front part of the neck with circular vibrating strokes, moving right down to the point where the sternum meets the clavicle. Go especially easy when moving over the Adam's apple and the windpipe, increasing the pressure in the less sensitive areas. Keep the pressure firm in these places and directed down toward the chest. Stroke lightly up to the point of origin and repeat

the movement twice.

10. Place the fingers of both hands at the lower borders of the trapezius and, using circular vibrating strokes, massage out toward the shoulders. For better reach, put the left hand on the right side of the neck and the right hand on the left side. Trace the muscle out to the tips of the shoulders, stroke firmly back in place and repeat the movement.

11. Now, beginning at the tops of the shoulders, stroke down in three-inch circles across the chest and abdominal area, tensing the muscles of the abdomen as you reach it. Keep the pressure heavy and directed toward the heart, exerting downward when above the heart and upward when below it. Move down to a point below the navel, then stroke up with the palms. Repeat the movement twice.

12. Perform vigorous petrissage on the pectoral muscles.

13. After this, perform the Swedish or cupped-hand version of tapotement on the pectorals, striking firmly and quickly.

14. Employing the cross-handed technique, reach under your armpits and perform petrissage on all parts of the latissimus dorsi that you can reach. Then move all the way down the sides of the chest through the ribcage to the tops of the hips, kneading the flesh between the thumbs and fingers. Stroke up to the point of origin, using the Swedish whiskbroom technique, and repeat the movement once or twice, depending upon your tolerance.

15. Place the heels of the hands at a point just under the navel. Stroke upward with deep pressure, moving up the abdominal area, ribcage and chest, crossing hands

above the chest and going out to the tops of the shoulders. Keep the pressure exerted toward the heart. Stroke lightly down to the point of origin and repeat the movement four or five times. Exert maximum pressure in this movement. Do the same movement on the right shoulder.

16. Place the palms flat against the sides of the neck and stroke down with deep pressure until the fingers reach the clavicle. Stroke lightly up and repeat this movement as long as it is comfortable.

17. Now move to the legs. Sit down and extend your legs as far as you can. Bend over and place the palms of both hands around the left or right ankle. Stroke up lightly to the groin. Stroke down to the point of origin, using the whiskbroom technique, and repeat the movement, increasing the pressure slightly. Repeat this movement four or five times until the pressure is fairly heavy.

18. Now place the thumbs of both hands adjacent to each other at the top of the anklebone, with the fingers resting lightly on either side. Using the circular vibrating technique, stroke upward with the fingers, pressing down with the thumbs and moving them only to change position. Move up to the groin in this manner, sliding down with the fingertips and repeating the movement once or twice, depending upon the time and comfort factors.

19. Grasp a point just above the ankle with the fingers of the right hand and take hold of the calf muscle with the fingers of the left. Perform petrissage on this muscle.

20. It is awkward to execute tapotement in this position, but you can try it, using the front part of the hands and striking with the wrist. If the movement cannot be performed cleanly, go on to the next treatment, which is:

21. Join both thumbs in the knee pit, with the fingers encircling the kneecap. Massage the kneecap and knee bone with circular vibrating strokes, pressing firmly with an upward direction.

22. Join the thumbs at the center of the foot on the instep. Knead the foot, pressing heavily and moving in small circles to the joints of the toes and back down to the bottom of the ankle. Knead the joints of the toes and balls of the feet with special concentration.

23. Place the heels of the hands on either side of the anklebone and stroke upward to the groin in three-inch circles. Keep the pressure heavy and in an upward direction. Repeat this once or twice.

24. Grasp the leg between the palms, the fingers resting just above the anklebone, and rub vigorously up the leg, producing as much friction as you can. Make a deep palmar stroke down to the original position and repeat this movement as many times as you wish.

25. Execute these same movements on the other leg.

26. Stand up. Bend over slightly to cause a slight protrusion of the buttocks. Perform petrissage on the buttocks with both hands, beginning at the top of the hips and moving up. Then grasp the buttocks between the palms and knead them firmly. End the series by stroking the buttocks with the whiskbroom movement, the fingers beginning at the tops of the hips and coming together at a spot just below the coccyx.

27. You cannot administer a whole-back massage to yourself, but you can reach those areas of the lower back which are most affected by poor posture and long periods spent in a sitting position. Join your thumbs at the small of your back. Stroke upward, using the circular vibrating

technique. When you can go no further, stroke lightly down to the original position, spread your thumbs apart slightly and begin again. Do this until you have covered as much of the back as you can.

If performed quickly and without a break, this entire treatment shouldn't take more than ten minutes. Of course if you have more time to devote to it, you can make your movements slower and more concentrated, and can stretch the massage out for as long a time as you wish. If you are pressed for time and only want to relieve a local ailment, you can use any one of these techniques alone. Remember, though, that some of them are immensely more effective when used in conjunction with other movements. Tapotement, for example, is an excellent reinforcement for petrissage. Deep stroking, also, should follow all fairly strenuous maneuvers to give the muscles a chance to relax.

FACIAL MASSAGE

Self-administered facial masssage can be performed any time during the day, but the optimum moment is at night before retiring. The muscles relax during slumber. If they have been properly conditioned before sleeping, they will relax into a new shape and tone.

Any of the techniques I described in the section on facial massage can be adapted for self-administration. For a more strictly cosmetic approach, you can use the following series of exercises:

1. Begin by placing your hands over your face, the fingertips resting slightly above the eyebrows. Applying pressure from the palms, stroke down, passing your fingertips over the eyes and stopping for a moment to

massage the eye sockets before traveling down the cheekbones to the chin. Bring the fingertips together at the tip of the chin and then resume the original position, repeating this movement as many times as you wish before going on to the next one.

2. Place the middle fingers of each hand below the earlobes. Stroke down in tiny circles, using the circular vibrating technique, moving along the jawline, just grazing it with the tips of your fingers. When your fingers have met at the jaw, stroke gently back to the point of origin. Now take a new position slightly below this. Stroke down again with your fingers meeting below the chin. Repeat these movements until you have covered the entire neck area and your fingers have come together at the meeting point of clavicle and sternum. Keep the pressure as heavy as you can bear and directed downward.

3. Now repeat this stroke around the facial area. Placing the index and middle fingers of both hands around the corners of the mouth, stroke upward in circular vibrating movements, moving over the cheekbones in a straight line to a point to the right of the temples. Slide down, take a new position and repeat the movement until you have massaged the entire facial area and the forehead.

4. Place your index fingers on both sides of your nose, slightly above the flares of the nostrils. Pressing down firmly, move up and along your cheekbones, around the eyes and on to the temples. Keep your mouth open and your facial muscles taut as you do this, so that you will be better able to follow the path of the bone. Stroke lightly down to the original position and perform this movement four or five times, until your face is tingling.

5. With the index and middle fingers of both hands

massage the forehead in slow circular vibrating strokes. Begin in the exact center and radiate outward. Then slide down to the bridge of the nose and knead the skin on either side. Knead all the way down the side of the nose, exerting upward pressure. Then stroke deeply around the corners of the mouth down to the chin. Exerting upward pressure, knead the flesh of the chin. Stroke up to the center of the forehead and perform the entire movement once or twice more.

6. Close your eyes and lightly stroke your eyelids, tracing a circular path around the lids and the sockets. This is an especially soothing maneuver, very good for insomnia and eyestrain headaches. Keep the pressure very light, just grazing the eyelids and increasing a bit around the sockets.

7. Incline your head slightly and let your facial muscles go loose. Perform petrissage on the facial muscles, working with the thumbs and forefingers on both sides of the face. Stroke down just beneath the chin and perform petrissage on the muscles lining the jaw.

8. Slap the face vigorously with the palms, striking rapidly and in unison on both sides of the face.

9. Repeat the first movement, deep stroking with the palms. Pretend that you are rubbing a healing balm into every pore and move slowly with downward pressure.

The facial massage can ease the burden of psychic troubles more effectively than any of the other massage movements. It is concentrated around the seats of the senses—the eyes, nose, mouth and lips—and can temporarily dispel minor anxieties. That is why it is most beneficial when done before bedtime. Try it. You may not even need a sleeping pill.

CHAPTER X

HOW TO CHOOSE A MASSEUR

The choice of a masseur, of course, is crucial.

The practice of massage is not restricted to the professional masseurs. It is used in various forms by many types of physical specialists and for many different reasons. Massage for relaxation, elementary conditioning and temporary relief of minor physical ills can be employed in the home by amateurs with much success. A thorough knowledge of the techniques I have described in this book plus a desire to please and relax the subject are all that is needed.

These techniques, however, are limited to normal people with the normal catalogue of aches, pains and anxieties. As I mentioned earlier, the amateur cannot massage away rheumatic or arthritic pain, severe muscle or ligament damage or psychotic disorder. These fields are reserved for specialists, working in special therapeutic environments with recourse to mechanical and chemical aids. A little learning can be a very dangerous thing in the gray area that separates ordinary massage from its more medical variations. When you have become proficient in the standard techniques, you still will not be qualified to perform physical therapy for even the most superficial ailment. People who respond well to massage tend to think of it as a panacea for all the world's ills and recommend it for everything from hangnail to heart disease. I would not want this book to further that impression.

If you need specialized massage, you will probably be advised of it. People with broken limbs on the mend are usually sent to physical therapists by their physicians. They undergo carefully structured treatments of massage, hydrotherapy and exercise. Do not apply self-massage if you happen to break or fracture a limb. You do not have the expertise or the equipment to do so. Let your doctor, working in cooperation with a physical therapist, assign a program of treatment for you. Do not offer to massage a friend who has suffered even a minor sprain. Injuries to the muscles and ligaments are very complicated. You need an X-ray to know exactly how they have affected the area and how they must be treated. A standard massage movement—like any one that I have described in this book—is too general to be employed in cases of injury.

Back injuries are still another area reserved for specialized massage. Notice I said *injuries,* not *pain.* There is a difference, as anyone who has suffered both can tell. Backaches from strain or exhaustion are temporary, involve no damage to the spine or the vertebrae, usually affect the muscles of the back, and will not worsen into any serious structural damage. Back injuries such as slipped discs, twisted sacroiliacs, etc., are extremely painful and ofttimes immobilizing. Under no circumstances should they be treated by anyone but a trained physician.

How do you know when a back pain is really a back injury? First, by the quality of the torment. If you cannot stand upright or stand at all; if the pain is almost intolerable, sharp and abrasive, not dull and throbbing like a muscle ache; if it is not ameliorated by massage, hot baths or muscle relaxers, go off to a doctor immediately. Also, if a back pain persists, not responding to any type of treatment, neither getting better nor worse, but staying on the same level for days and weeks on end, there might be structural damage in the making. In cases like this a massage might be the straw that breaks your back. A good orthopedist is a much better idea.

Chiropractors practice a form of massage. Their techniques are unique and are predicated upon the theory that the spine is the seat of almost all illness. Their profession is controversial because of the outlandishness of this theory and also because the taint of quackery has long been attached to it. Chiropractors are not doctors of medicine. They can hang out shingles and call themselves doctors after having been graduated from a school of chiropractic and being licensed by the state. These requirements are not very stringent, and many unscrupulous, totally fraudulent practitioners have entered the ranks by fulfilling them. There are also many more dedicated chiropractors, who do not make wild claims for their science, but do insist that their manipulations ease pain, correct deformity and often spare the necessity of surgery.

In spite of their ambiguous reputations, chiropractors do a flourishing business. Many people who do physical labor swear by them. Dancers and acrobats—who, in addition to exerting their bodies, stretch and contort them into unnatural positions—often make weekly and sometimes daily visits for "adjustments" or repositionings of those out-of-place muscles. I have spoken to people who claim that their slipped discs were ameliorated by regular visits, others who claim that migraine headaches and sexual impotency were cured and even one person who swears that an inch was added to his height. In the face of all this personal testimony it would be unfair to condemn the entire profession out of hand. I have also spoken to people who reported no benefit from the chiropractic treatment, and some who said it even worsened their symptons. If you contemplate going to a chiropractor, you'll have to make up your own mind as to the efficacy of the treatment.

There are certain ways of ascertaining the integrity and worth of a chiropractor. Equipment and environment are important considerations. If the chiropractor has a professional office, no different in appearance from that of a medical doctor's, complete with nurse, magazines (Muzak is optional) and multitudes of patients, you can guess that a certain amount of financial success has been achieved. The chiropractor does not have a captive audience as does the medical doctor. He thrives on the good results he produces and the word of mouth of his satisfied patients. The reputable chiropractor has a treatment room with a revolving couch, separate from his office. He does not use a massage table, and he does not place the patients on the floor. The patient either sits or lies on the couch while the ministrations are being performed. The chiropractor also has a little meter with a probe attached to it with which he measures the heat being generated around the base of the neck and top of the spine. This helps him determine how far and in what manner the spine is out of line.

The good chiropractor never performs manipulations without first having X-rays taken. Conscious of his tenuous hold on respectability, he usually goes over the X-rays with the patient, pointing out the area of dislocation and explaining how his treatment will correct it. He prescribes a different frequency of visits for varying stages in the therapeutic procedure, lessening the frequency as the treatment progresses, until the patient usually has to return only several times a year for periodic adjustments. The chiropractor does a good deal of explaining to protect himself from the charge of misrepresentation. Thus you can know quite a bit about the healer you've chosen and can make an educated decision on his merits before committing yourself to a course of treatment.

The best place for a relaxing, mildly therapeutic massage is in the home, under the expert hands of someone with whom you are intimate and affectionate. But the home is not and never can be a gymnasium. If you want a complete conditioning regimen, the facilities of the health club are the only answer.

There are many to choose from and more springing up every day as the demand increases. There are several criteria which should guide you in deciding which club to join.

1. Facilities. It is pointless to limit yourself. There are

so many clubs that have complete facilities that there is no reason to join one which doesn't. A swimming pool and some form of sauna bath are absolute musts, as are a massage room and an exercise area. Facilities like basketball, handball, tracks, etc., are nice extras for the sports-minded, but can be dispensed with for those who are interested in sharpening body tone, not athletic skills.

2. Staff. A health club must be adequately staffed. In addition to the various pool, bath and locker attendants, there must also be trained people to see to your physical conditioning. Licensed masseurs, gymnastic and calisthenic coaches and swimming coaches are always available in a good health club.

3. Cleanliness. A health club must be spotless. A speck of dirt in an area where the body is so vulnerable is equal to the entire contents of a filthy city street. Pool water should be regularly changed, as should the pads on the massage tables, the towels, etc. The steam baths should be thoroughly cleaned and disinfected. There should be a pleasant, nondeodorant smell about the place. The smell of cleanliness.

Most health clubs have a membership plan whereby you pay a certain sum for a specified amount of visits, or you buy a year's membership. Shop around very carefully before you settle on one, or you might find yourself trapped in an unpleasant environment.

Exercise can be a lonely business. If you are just beginning to attend a health club on a regular basis, it might be wise to do so with a close friend. A routinized physical regimen can become a bore to people who have not totally incorporated it into their daily lives. You might be too lazy or tired to exert the necessary energy to get there and go through all the necessary procedures. The conditioning process does not have instant results. You may become discouraged if you don't notice a dramatic change within a couple of weeks. And you won't, although if you can stick it out for a few months, you will see the difference. It will be much easier to share these first demanding months with someone else. You can take turns encouraging each other, buoying each other's dragging spirits. The tedium of some exercises will be lightened by this company, the early stages of the conditioning process will be much more fun, and you'll both probably last until the exercise itself becomes enjoyable and necessary to you.

Taking care of yourself is a demanding chore. Most people have to force themselves by an effort of will out of their sedentary lives into more healthful activity. Exercise is exhausting. It takes time for the body to learn to like it. Give yourself that time. You won't regret it.

All the reputable health clubs have one or two licensed masseurs on the premises. There are levels of quality between them as there are in every other profession. A good masseur must be immaculate, with trimmed, clean fingernails and soft, smooth hands and no offending perfume or body odor. The good masseur has the uncanny ability to make his or her whole body and personality vanish, leaving only a pair of strong, gentle, ministering hands. The good masseur is a listener, not a talker. He does not try to impose his personality on the subject; he never discusses his personal life, asks advice or tries to establish a personal relationship. As far as his technical ability goes, you will be the best judge of that. Just as you know immediately when you're in a car with a good driver or in a chair with a good dentist or barber, so you'll know whether or not you're being treated by a competent masseur.

The practice of massage has become so popular that now you can get masseurs who make house calls. Newspapers and magazines are full of classified advertisements for traveling masseurs. The range of choice is fairly wide among them. There are male and female, licensed and unlicensed, massage teams of two women, two men or a man and a woman, and other combinations which, if nothing else, would make for a very crowded living room. Choosing a masseur in this fashion is a slightly speculative venture, but there are some guidelines you can follow.

1. Choose a masseur of the same sex. If you are interested in an erotic adventure, you can go in any direction you wish, but if you want a serious massage, it must be given by someone of the same sex.

2. Choose a licensed masseur. Anyone can place an ad in the paper claiming to be an unlicensed masseur. No training or certification is necessary; all you need do is call yourself one and you can hang out a shingle. Unfortunately, I can give you that piece of advice from personal experience. My first massage in America was by a man. It was the shortest in my entire life. I went screaming out of his deserted studio about ten seconds after it had started.

In order to be licensed a masseur must finish a course of study at one of the many accredited massage schools, pass a test and be certified by the state. The license is no guarantee of competence or even of respectability, but chances are that a licensed masseur is much more competent and respectable than an unlicensed one.

If you are choosing from newspaper ads, without recommendation or previous acquaintance, call several masseurs and ask about their backgrounds, prices, availability, etc. Don't be in a hurry to make a final decision. A home massage can cost anywhere from ten to thirty-five dollars an hour; it's a costly investment and should be carefully considered.

A masseur's price is no indication of ability. The price is simply predicated on what the market will bear. In affluent suburbs where there are fewer masseurs per capita, massage can cost a good deal more than it's worth, whereas in urban areas where competition among masseurs is intense, you can get the best professional service at a very reasonable price.

One can usually measure the difference between a necessity and a luxury by the price. In New York City a massage costs roughly from $7.50 to $10, but in Sweden the price is about $1.50. My mother spends relatively little on hairdos and cosmetics, but she would never go without her weekly massage.

Reading this book may have given you an interest in pursuing massage as a career. If so, do not stop here. The movements, procedures and conditions described in this book are meant primarily for the massage of intimate by intimate. You have a lot more to learn if you want to start making a living as a masseur.

You should master all the techniques of massage. The best way to do this is to enroll in an accredited school of massage. The yellow pages of your phone book can give you a wide choice. In addition to massage these schools teach anatomy and give an elementary grounding in physical therapeutic procedures. Professional certification differs in each state, but they will not be impossibly rigorous if you are properly trained.

The information in this book is more than sufficient to make you a good unlicensed masseur. You can bring relaxation and happiness to close friends and loved ones by being an enthusiastic masseur and an appreciative subject. There is nothing like a massage to provide the emotional cement for a new relationship or to rekindle feelings of trust and affection in an old one. Remember, no matter what the conditions are, massage is a transmission of love and should always be approached in that way.